5-Minute Mindfulness for Pregnancy

5-MINUTE
Mindfulness
for Pregnancy

Simple Practices to Feel Calm, Present, and Connected to Your Baby

Josephine Atluri

ROCKRIDGE PRESS

For general information on our other products and services, please contact our Customer Care Department within the United States at (866) 744-2665, or outside the United States at (510) 253-0500.

Paperback ISBN: 978-1-63878-341-1 | eBook ISBN: 978-1-63878-539-2

Manufactured in the United States of America

Interior and Cover Designer: Jenny Paredes
Art Producer: Alyssa Williams
Editor: Eun H. Jeong
Production Manager: Jose Olivera

All illustrations used under license from Shutterstock.com

0 1 2 3 4 5 6 7 8 9 10

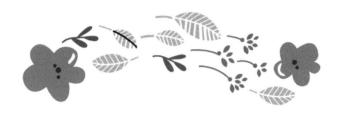

For Josephine & Juliette ~
our latest embodiment of love.
For Pramod ~
the catalyst for the manifestation of my dreams.

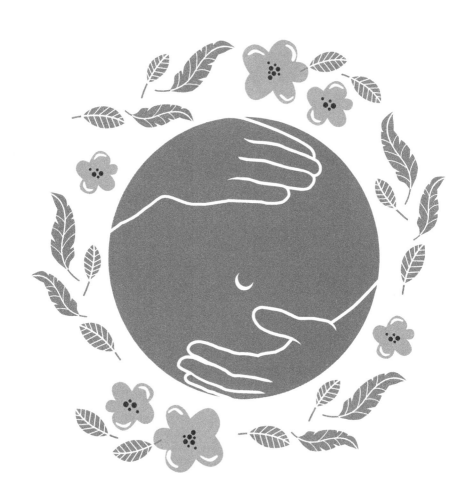

Contents

Introduction

Congratulations on your pregnancy! Whether this is your first time being pregnant or you've done this before, you're entering a vibrant season of life filled with so many unique experiences that you will likely cherish forever. As you witness your baby's miraculous development, you will also undergo significant changes to your physical appearance, your perspective, and your life overall. All of these experiences make for an unforgettable time of anticipation and profound feelings.

However exciting, all of this change can be a lot to navigate, and it can impact your well-being. So, while ensuring your baby's healthy growth, it's also essential to care for yourself throughout your pregnancy journey. Your fitness, nutrition, and physical health are important, of course. However, your mental and emotional well-being also play a major role in both your health and the development and delivery of your baby. Every kindness you extend to yourself will benefit both you and your baby, including giving yourself compassion and time to rest and reflect.

As a mother of seven children (I have been pregnant several times, adopted, and also partnered with two surrogates to carry four of our children), I remember how challenging it was to cherish the gestational experience. For my first three children, I was preoccupied with worries about my pregnancy and

the future, so much so that I felt overwhelmed and unable to be present in my journey. Looking back, I wish I'd had the tools to care for myself so I could have enjoyed being pregnant, an unmatched experience that took several heartbreaking years of assisted reproductive therapy to finally come to fruition.

Many years later, after discovering meditation and mindfulness for myself and then becoming certified to teach others these skills, I was able to apply mindfulness to our later pregnancies. As a result, I noticed marked differences in my pregnancy experiences. I finally savored the process! I also improved my overall state of being through reduced stress and increased positivity. These personal experiences fueled my passion to help other people on their path to parenthood by showing them how to incorporate mindfulness into their own journeys.

If you're new to mindfulness, here's a brief overview: Mindfulness is a keen awareness of the present moment, achieved by paying attention to oneself, one's environment, and one's interactions with others. Mindfulness is done without judgment, meaning that you don't judge thoughts or experiences—you just notice them and let them pass by. When you apply mindfulness as the foundation for your daily activities, you begin to experience life through a lens of intention, awareness,

possibility, and appreciation. Even after your very first attempt, mindfulness can bring a sense of joy, ease, and presence into your life. By applying awareness on a daily basis, you'll feel increasingly able to navigate challenges, fortifying your courage, strength, and resilience.

Given the many benefits of mindfulness, I am inspired to empower expecting parents with the tools and strategies to enhance their well-being and handle whatever comes their way during pregnancy with confidence and grace.

This book contains a wide variety of easy-to-follow exercises that can be practiced in just five minutes, making it an approachable way to access presence on a daily basis. Within that short time frame, these exercises will open the door to reflection, serenity, positivity, and connection with yourself and your baby.

While mindfulness is an effective activity for navigating the pregnancy transformation, if you ever experience any exceedingly debilitating feelings such as depression or anxiety, please seek the support of a medical professional. This book should not replace medical treatment or guidance. Perinatal depression and anxiety occur during many pregnancies. There is no shame in seeking extra support when needed. See page 154 for resources for professional help.

As you embark on this adventure, I encourage you to approach each day gently and with self-compassion. It takes time to build a new habit and adjust to an alternative way of thinking. Remember that you are brave for stepping out of your comfort zone and being vulnerable to this introspective process. Your daily efforts will translate into a richer experience of yourself, your pregnancy journey, and the present moment. Starting your mindfulness exploration now, during your pregnancy, is a great first step to intentional living that you can carry on well into parenthood.

How to Use This Book

The exercises in this book each take just five minutes to complete, enabling you to quickly reap the benefits of mindfulness for your overall well-being. The best way to cultivate and sustain a new habit is consistency, so try to practice daily. Experiment with different times of day. When you find something that works with your schedule, hold yourself accountable by adding your practice to your calendar, like any other appointment. If you miss a session, however, don't feel bad. New habits often require adjustment periods. The most important thing is to go at your own pace.

Part 1 of this book explores the core principles of mindfulness, its overall benefits, and its positive applications during pregnancy. Part 2 consists of eight chapters with a variety of mindfulness practices. These practices target the mind, body, connection with the baby, difficult emotions, uncertainty, support systems, and daily habits. You'll do this through different activities, including meditation, visualization, breathing exercises, gentle movement, journaling, and awareness exercises. We'll explore these in more detail in chapter 1.

It can be helpful to have a timer set for five minutes to keep you on track. For example, in journaling sessions, you can choose one prompt from a multi-prompt exercise to work on

for five minutes and answer the other prompts on other days if you prefer. As you become more comfortable with the practices and desire longer sessions, simply extend your time or combine several practices.

When you begin the exercises, start where you are and give yourself grace. Approach each exercise with patience for yourself and the process. Try to let go of any expectations and give yourself permission to deeply experience any shifts that occur from this new exploration. You may encounter moments of vulnerability as you step out of your comfort zone. Each time you try again, however, you reignite your resolve, courage, strength, and commitment to this beautiful awakening.

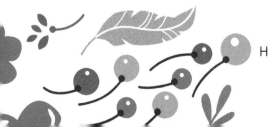

PART ONE

An Introduction to Mindfulness

In this first part of the book, you'll explore various ways to cultivate mindfulness, or present-moment awareness, in order to nurture yourself and enrich your experiences. You will also gain a strong understanding of the impact that daily mindfulness practices can have on your life, such as awakening your connection to your authentic self and the world around you.

After learning how the power of mindfulness can expand your consciousness and enhance your everyday life, you'll discover how you can apply mindfulness to your pregnancy journey. More than anything, tuning in to the present moment elevates the transformative process of creating a life. Lastly, before we delve into the actual 5-minute exercises that you can do on a daily basis, the final section of part 1 will provide practical tips on how to successfully weave a mindfulness practice into your life in a sustainable way.

CHAPTER 1

Practicing Mindfulness 101

In this chapter, we will cover the basics of mindfulness: a basic description, a brief overview of the origins of mindfulness, and its applications in everyday life. This section will highlight the various types of mindfulness that you'll encounter in this book and the benefits of cultivating a practice. Mindfulness is often heralded for its ability to resolve stress and anxiety, but there are many other benefits of tapping into awareness that we will explore.

If this is your first foray into mindfulness and you feel apprehensive about your ability to follow along, you're not alone. Mindfulness can feel challenging at first because it isn't something we are necessarily taught in our childhood. Plus, the busyness of daily life can keep us distracted and disconnected. We'll address some common challenges that can get in the way of mindfulness, and you'll learn ways to circumvent these potential issues.

This chapter will introduce the keys to building a consistent mindfulness practice that you can enjoy for years to come.

What Is Mindfulness?

Mindfulness is a purposeful awareness of the present moment without judgment. It is an awareness of oneself physically, mentally, and emotionally. Mindfulness is the ability to witness your own environment and your interactions with others as a present-moment observer, absorbing all of the sensory experiences as they come.

Mindfulness can be thought of as the foundation upon which every other aspect of life builds. For example, when you cultivate awareness, you can be mindful when you eat, work, exercise, or talk to friends and family. Oftentimes, we get caught up in the chaos of life, in ruminations about the past and worries over the uncertainty of the future, and we run on autopilot. Conversely, when we are mindful, we are consciously connecting to the world around us with open-mindedness instead of missing out on life's joys due to distractions.

Living in the present moment enhances your overall experience, but it has been found that mindfulness can also change your brain structure and, with that, its functionality! Numerous research studies have used MRI technology to see the effects of mindfulness and meditation on the brain. They found the gray matter in the prefrontal cortex grew, while the amygdala shrank over the course of weeks and months of practicing mindfulness. The prefrontal cortex is responsible for cognition and decision-making, whereas the amygdala is associated with emotions like fear and anxiety. Thus, mindfulness increases the ability to handle emotions from a place of logic and clarity, which can greatly impact the quality of your life.

What Mindfulness Isn't

There are many misconceptions about mindfulness that should be debunked before we get started. First, many people think that mindfulness is synonymous with meditation. In actuality, mindfulness can be thought of as the overarching framework in which there are various techniques, including meditation. Meditations are included in this book, but if you have difficulty meditating, there are many other exercises provided that you can do to practice and achieve mindfulness.

Another misconception is that mindfulness involves complex steps, postures, or poses, and that you need special equipment like meditation pillows, incense, or candles. On the contrary, you'll find that mindfulness can be as simple as observing your breath. Nothing is required but you.

The Origins and Evolution of Mindfulness

Mindfulness has been around for thousands of years, with origins rooted in Eastern religions. In Hinduism, both scriptures and yoga make references to a state of enlightenment achieved through meditative consciousness, or *samadhi*. Those familiar with yoga have experienced the final pose in the practice called *savasana*, which is a resting pose meant to relax the mind and body and invite present-moment awareness and grounding. Mindfulness and meditation also have roots in Buddhism, as the practice of being mindful of the self is one of the major tenets of the Buddha's eightfold path guiding followers on a journey toward awakening.

Mindfulness later evolved into its own standalone practice in Western cultures, popularized by authorities like Jon Kabat-Zinn, Zindel Segal, Mark Williams, and John Teasdale and backed with scientific legitimacy from neuroscientists like Dr. Sara Lazar. Kabat-Zinn developed the Mindfulness-Based Stress Reduction program (MBSR), which is an eight-week program that helps people manage their pain, stress, depression, and anxiety via mindfulness, meditation, and cognitive therapy.

Mindfulness-Based Cognitive Therapy (MBCT), created by Segal, Williams, and Teasdale, helps people with chronic mood disorders and unhappiness become more aware of their behaviors in order to change their relationship with their thoughts. In addition to these widely recognized mindfulness programs, numerous research studies back the benefits of mindfulness from both a physical and psychological perspective. The common theme in this research is that mindfulness has the potential to help a person decrease stress, reduce side effects of mood disorders and pain from illness, and achieve general improvement in overall health.

Types of Mindfulness

The beauty of mindfulness is that there are many paths to achieving awareness that can address your specific needs. These include meditation, visualization, breathwork, gentle movement, journaling, and general awareness exercises—all of which we will address in this book. Each of these techniques involves the art of consciously connecting to the present moment. The only difference is in the execution.

Some days you'll feel inspired to sit in silence and just breathe, while other days you'll be drawn toward mindful movement. A process that may work for you most days may not be effective on another day. Just pay attention to how you are feeling and determine the process that feels appropriate at that time. The more you practice mindfulness, the more you'll feel in tune with your needs.

Meditation

Like mindfulness, meditation is a wellness practice that has been around for thousands of years in Eastern cultures. It has gained increased popularity over the years in Western society, as meditation not associated with religion made it more accessible to a broader audience. Meditation is essentially a way of training the brain to be aware and observe the present moment without judgment. Sometimes it involves a point of focus, like your breath, or a vehicle to stay grounded in the present, such as a mantra or positive affirmation like "I am calm." We will explore many types of meditations in this book, from body scans to walking meditations and more, which will give you the opportunity to vary your point of focus.

Visualization

Visualization is the process of imagining experiences and outcomes in vivid detail. One purpose of visualization is to open your mind up to possibilities that may otherwise seem out of reach. When you imagine a journey in your mind, you picture yourself going through the process and also feeling the emotions so you can feel confident in replicating those steps in real life. Over time, this vision will feel attainable. Visualization also cultivates calm, making it a beneficial mindfulness practice. This calmness can come from visualizing yourself in a peaceful place or imagining yourself doing something in a composed manner.

Breathwork

Breathwork is another mindfulness approach that keeps you grounded in the present moment. Numerous techniques can help you manipulate your breath, such as counting varied lengths of time, changing the speed and pace of your breath, and varying the location from where the breath originates. Breathwork is a powerful mindfulness tool for two reasons: First, slowing down your breath sends a signal to your brain that you are moving from a state of stress to calm. Secondly, following a pattern of breathing requires you to focus on your breath in the present moment. By following a pattern, it becomes difficult to ruminate over things in the past or worry about the future. Breathing exercises can serve as a standalone practice or the foundation for a meditation in which your point of focus is your breath.

Check with your healthcare provider to see if you should follow any safety guidelines before starting any breathing exercise. Discontinue if you feel light-headed, dizzy, or anxious.

Gentle Movement

Can you be mindful while moving your body? Absolutely! A common misconception is that mindfulness requires you to be still in order to clear your mind. However, there are no rules against coupling mindfulness with movement, and this certainly does not inhibit awareness. In fact, gentle exercises done mindfully can strengthen the mind-body connection. When you activate your body slowly and with intention, you can witness what is happening in the present and reflect on how each movement makes your body feel. By creating a connection between your mind and your body, gentle movement can have positive repercussions in your daily activities.

Journaling

Journaling is a cathartic and effective mindfulness exercise that doesn't require you to learn anything new, making it one of the quickest ways to tap into your awareness. In this book, the journaling exercises use prompts or questions to invite you to reflect, which will lead to insights about yourself and your relationship with others. You can also journal without a prompt by simply recording down whatever flows out of you, whether it be in a notebook, on your computer or phone, or into a voice recording program. In this open format, the journaling can be used for spontaneous thoughts, ideas, or dreams, or even as a "brain dump," where you can offload anything weighing on your mind that may be bothersome or stressful.

This practice of letting go is an effective way of navigating overwhelming emotions.

Awareness Exercises

Another way of accessing mindfulness is through general awareness exercises. Essentially, an awareness exercise encourages you to perform a seemingly ordinary task, such as walking, and combine it with mindfulness prompts to deepen your experience of the present-moment activity. For example, a walking awareness exercise would challenge you to tune in to all your senses as you go for a stroll, enabling you to fully connect to the beauty of life in real time. Awareness exercises can push you to experience life through a new perspective and enrich moments that you might otherwise take for granted or simply not notice.

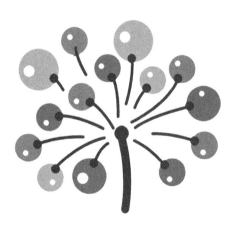

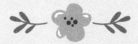

COME AS YOU ARE

This book recognizes that all fertility journeys are different. There are various ways that people reach the point of pregnancy, just as there are many paths to parenthood. If you experienced a difficult journey before finally becoming pregnant, please know that these exercises are inclusive of your unique needs. The beauty of mindfulness is that the exercises meet you where you are at in your personal process, free of judgment. If you have experienced any trauma on your path to parenthood, these introspective exercises will give you a safe space to dig deep and heal. If you are new to mindfulness and feel apprehensive about your ability to follow along, just know that these exercises are designed to be approachable and manageable. If you are feeling stress and anxiety during this time of life, consider this resource as your partner in navigating those challenges in a thoughtful way. It bears repeating that if any feelings become overwhelming, it is brave and effective to seek help from a mental health professional.

If you are part of the LGBTQ+ or nonbinary communities, please know that you are seen and represented here. With no exceptions, this book aims to provide everyone with a place where you can explore yourself and your unique relationships, and clearly tune in to your pregnancy journey in preparation for the beautiful transition into parenthood.

The Benefits of Mindfulness

Pregnancy is a complicated journey because of all the mixed emotions and changes that occur. Practicing mindfulness exercises during this season of your life will benefit you both in the present moment and the long run, as you transition into your new role as a parent and beyond. Your pregnancy is a great time to start practicing mindfulness, because it will help you live in the "now" and appreciate the beauty of what's happening as you and your baby develop. Mindfulness will also help you manage any stress, anxiety, or heavy feelings that may emerge during various stages of pregnancy. Tapping into your awareness can help you shift from a state of negativity to one of positivity that can translate into increased gratitude, compassion, love, and joy.

Live in the Present

In today's society, we are constantly inundated with information and stretched by all of our obligations. It's not a surprise that staying present in the moment has become foreign to most of us. It can be easy to get stuck in a habit of ruminating over the past and looking ahead to the future, which brings us out of living in the moment. The beauty of mindfulness is that it gives us a way to stay tethered to the present. When you utilize techniques like meditation and breathwork, your focus moves to something happening right now, such as watching your breath, repeating a mantra, or simply being your authentic self.

Manage Fear, Stress, and Anxiety

Stress, anxiety, and fear can bubble up when you dwell on past experiences, fixate on the future, or brood over uncertainty. Mulling over past mistakes, for example, can make you feel bad about yourself, and these negative thoughts and feelings can lead to stress. Similarly, thinking about all the things you have to do or imagining future scenarios creates feelings of uncertainty and overwhelm, which breed angst. By incorporating mindfulness into your daily life, you can become attuned to your disposition and notice when you start to shift into negativity. From this place of awareness, you can acknowledge those feelings and then respond with calming mindfulness techniques. For example, if you notice physical symptoms of stress showing up in your body, you can apply gentle movement exercises like prenatal yoga to alleviate your discomfort.

Release Judgment

One benefit of harnessing awareness is the ability to identify and reframe your relationships with difficult emotions like judgment. We all have an innate negativity bias; as a result, it's common for us to judge ourselves and others. Through mindfulness, you'll notice your tendencies and learn to challenge their validity. In the process, you might uncover deeper narratives or beliefs that unconsciously impact your life. The process of observing your patterns of thoughts and emotions enables you to release judgments that prevent you from being at peace with your authentic self and seeking out new possibilities.

Develop Greater Self-Compassion and Self-Love and Improve Self-Confidence

When we tap into awareness of ourselves, we begin to witness how we treat ourselves in the moment. We're not typically conscious of the thoughts that we allow our inner critic to have about the way we look, feel, and live. Have you ever passed a mirror and criticized your reflection? Incorporating awareness into your self-talk can highlight your self-perception and, with consistent effort over time, can change how you treat yourself. Consciousness can lead to greater self-love and self-compassion, especially when paired with mindfulness strategies like positive affirmations. In fact, studies have shown that using strategies like affirmations can actually rewire your brain, creating positive changes and increased feelings of self-worth. When you shower yourself with more love and compassion, you begin to recognize your inner beauty, and in turn, improve your self-esteem and self-confidence.

Shift from Negativity to Positivity

Another benefit of mindfulness is the ability to recognize the need to shift from a state of negativity to one of positivity. As you go throughout your day, you may encounter triggers that cause you to feel upset or less than. Once you've entered that frame of mind, it can be easy to get sucked into a spiral of negative thoughts and, before you know it, trapped in a web of gloom. By practicing awareness of your thoughts and feelings, you can identify negativity and implement strategies that work toward a more positive perspective. Plus, by harnessing your awareness abilities, you may begin to notice patterns in your reactions and understand your triggers. Understanding your patterns of behavior and what triggers you gives you the ability to prevent or diffuse negativity.

Cultivate Gratitude and Joy

When you live in the moment, you tend to be aware of everything around you and all that you have. You also become attuned to everything that's happening in real time, instead of in retrospect. This consciousness enables you to cultivate gratitude and joy because you open yourself to life as it's happening, versus being tethered to the past or future. Over time, rooting yourself in mindfulness can enhance your ability to look at life through a lens of genuine joy and consistent gratitude.

The Challenges of Mindfulness

While some aspects of mindfulness can seem simple and straightforward in theory, putting the concepts into actual practice can pose challenges. A common issue is the idea that you can't turn off your thoughts. Or the thoughts themselves might feel so overwhelming that you feel even more anxious when you sit down and acknowledge them.

Another challenge is thinking that you're not doing the exercises correctly because they aren't meeting your expectations. Plus, in a world where multitasking is revered, practicing a singular conscious presence might feel difficult or counterintuitive, and makes you feel unaccomplished.

All of these concerns are valid. Mindfulness is a new way of approaching life, so it will take time to unlearn old ways of thinking and adopt alternative approaches. Fortunately, the information and exercises in this book will gently guide and support you in your exploration of awareness. Next, we'll cover how to navigate these and other prevalent challenges in order to realize an enriching mindfulness practice.

Learning to Sit with Ourselves Is Hard

For many, running around due to overly scheduled lives has become an acceptable way to operate. Therefore, the idea of sitting with yourself to tap into awareness and calm can seem foreign and even daunting. Maybe it feels contrary to what you think is an effective way to address your true feelings. However, it is in the quiet and slower-paced moments that you can actually hear what is going on inside and achieve clarity.

Remember to take things slow, especially with the demands of pregnancy, and ease into this new mindset with grace. Also, take turns with the various types of exercises presented in this book. By varying your awareness efforts, you won't get stuck trying to make something work that may not feel natural yet.

Difficult Emotions and Feelings May Come to Light

Many people live in a constant state of activity, and some scurry through life as a coping mechanism for avoiding difficult emotions and issues. Cultivating awareness through breathwork, meditation, visualization, and journaling requires tuning in to yourself in the moment. This intentional reflection can stir up difficult feelings, memories, or concerns that you may have been working so hard to avoid, especially if you've had a challenging path to pregnancy or other past issues. As a result, you could start to feel anxious and fearful. However frightening these thoughts may feel, they are completely normal when facing big emotions. It's important not to judge your experience. One good way to handle difficult emotions or anxiety is to label your thoughts when they come up. Depending on what it is, you can label the disturbing thought as a worry, a task, a sensation, a sound, or a want. The process of labeling can remind you that it's just a thought. It does not inform your identity. This realization can reduce the impact of the thought on your mental well-being.

Our Minds Like to Wander

People have *thousands* of thoughts on any given day. With that many thoughts floating in and out of your mind, the idea of focusing your attention on one thing happening in the present moment can feel intimidating! To relieve the pressure to clear your mind, remember that it's perfectly normal for our minds to wander and for thoughts to pop up, even when we are trying so hard to be fully present. Rather than fixating on preventing a wandering mind, view your mindfulness efforts as a chance to practice handling your thoughts and interruptions, as that is what happens in everyday life. As you practice mindfulness, when a thought enters your mind, gently acknowledge it and continue with the mindfulness practice without placing any judgment on the thought or yourself.

We Are Prone to Multitasking

The ability to multitask is often heralded as a positive attribute because of the idea that you can get a lot more done in less time. Plus, multitasking can feel like the best option when you have a never-ending to-do list, especially with a baby on the way. One downside of multitasking, however, is that your focus gets spread out over multiple things at once, making it impossible to be fully present with any of the tasks you are juggling. Research shows that when you focus your attention on one thing at a time, you can accomplish tasks individually with greater concentration and success. And chances are, you can achieve that single task more quickly because you aren't getting distracted by other things.

"I Don't Think I'm Doing It Right"

A question I hear often when I teach meditation and mindfulness is "Am I doing this right?" When we attempt anything new, we often have expectations for how the experience should play out and what we should achieve. The best way to approach mindfulness is to be open to possibilities and allow the experience to unfold organically. There isn't a right way to be mindful or to meditate. Each experience will be different, person to person, day to day, depending on your mood and other circumstances. Despite any differences in experiences, every time you attempt to meditate or be mindful, you're making progress just by trying. Every attempt at accessing awareness gives your brain valuable practice.

Mindfulness Can Make Us Sleepy

Another valid concern is that you may fall asleep while doing a mindfulness exercise like meditating. Perhaps this has already happened to you in the past. When doing any mindfulness exercise, everything about the experience is an opportunity to unearth something that needs to be addressed. In some cases it's deeply buried emotions that have been avoided. In other instances, exhaustion is what comes to the surface. If you meditate and find yourself falling asleep every now and then, it's okay. Your ability to fall asleep at that moment means that you have fully surrendered to the practice, and that's great news! During various stages of pregnancy, you will naturally feel more tired than usual. If you find it happening too often, change positions or try one of the more active mindfulness exercises in the book.

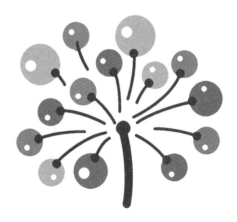

STRUGGLING WITH MINDFULNESS? THESE TIPS CAN HELP

L earning to sit with yourself can feel hard, especially if you've never taken a moment to just be with yourself without being busy. Here are a few more tips to set yourself up for a successful introduction to mindfulness:

Let go of expectations. Expectations of the process and outcomes can create disappointment and stress. Instead, try your best to be flexible and flow with what happens, much like water flowing around obstacles in its path. You'll find a great deal of freedom in the process of letting go.

Remember that you are not your thoughts. It bears reminding that thoughts will happen and that's okay! You do not need to identify with your thoughts. Your thoughts do not define you. Allow them to pop up, and acknowledge them without judgment. Label the thought if that helps you detach from it. Then let the thought go and return to your practice.

Breathe it out. If something overwhelming comes to the surface during any mindfulness practice, try to sit with it and understand why it came up for you. While doing so, incorporate one of the breathing techniques covered in this book, such as Square Breathing (page 40), to help move yourself from a state of stress to calm.

Building a Consistent Practice Takes Time

Carving out five minutes to practice mindfulness can feel like a lot. And like any new habit, it will take time, patience, and practice in order to build a routine. But later, when you add all the 5-minute sessions together, you will realize a wealth of results.

One of the best ways to ensure success is to pair your new habit with an existing habit that you do consistently every day. For example, if you already have a nightly bedtime routine that you do diligently, try pairing your 5-minute mindfulness exercise with your established ritual, either before or after. It can feel a lot easier to schedule a new habit in this manner rather than trying to find a whole new time slot in what may already be a busy day. The goal of your new mindfulness routine is to consistently cultivate calm and awareness. Consider each 5-minute exercise a small step toward the bigger goal of becoming a more present person—and there's no time like pregnancy to start making that a priority.

The Power of Five Minutes

We've mentioned five minutes a lot here. That's because a good way to ensure the success of your mindfulness practice is to keep it short and simple. Whenever you introduce a new habit into your life, it's easiest to start off small so it feels manageable and accessible, and then gradually expand your practice. The exercises in this book are all things that you can do within five minutes and quickly reap powerful benefits such as increased calm and decreased stress. It may seem inconceivable to accomplish something beneficial in such a short amount of time. However, we do it all the time—brushing our teeth, reading an article, talking to a loved one. All of these things can take just a few minutes, and yet they are still productive moments in our day. The significance of a 5-minute practice is that you can always find time to fit it into your day, no matter how busy it may be.

Key Takeaways

Congratulations! You have taken the first step to building a consistent mindfulness practice. Here are the key takeaways covered in this first chapter:

✦ Mindfulness is a purposeful awareness of the present moment without judgment. It is the foundation upon which every other aspect of life builds.

✦ Mindfulness helps us become cognizant of our actions, such as when we start to do too many things at once, causing stress and overwhelm.

✦ There are many approaches to achieving awareness that can address your particular needs, such as meditation, visualization, breathwork, gentle movement, journaling, and general awareness exercises. Each of these techniques involves the art of consciously connecting to the present moment. The only difference is in the execution.

✦ Benefits of mindfulness include managing stress, fear, and anxiety; living in the present; releasing judgment; developing self-compassion, self-love, and self-confidence; shifting from negativity to positivity; and cultivating gratitude and joy.

✦ Although challenges to mindfulness exist, there isn't one right way to practice mindfulness.

✦ If you release your expectations of what should happen and become open to possibilities, you'll have a smoother experience.

✦ You can create a sustainable mindfulness practice through consistency, by pairing this new habit with an existing ritual, and by starting off with small time frames for practicing.

You are giving yourself such an amazing gift by choosing to embrace and incorporate mindfulness into your life during this time of transition. By keeping in mind these takeaways, you'll be prepared to embark on a remarkable path of growth. Next, let's explore more about how and why to weave mindfulness into your pregnancy journey.

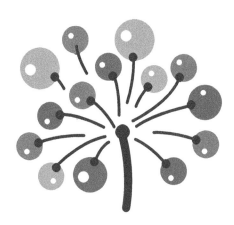

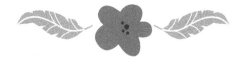

CHAPTER 2

Mindfulness for Pregnancy

Now that you've learned the basics of mindfulness and how a daily practice can positively impact your well-being, let's explore how mindfulness can be especially beneficial during the gestational period. Mindfulness practices have the ability to decrease stress and anxiety during pregnancy, which can positively affect your well-being and the development of your baby in utero. Practicing mindfulness harnesses your inner calm, allowing you to regulate your emotions, even in the thick of complicated feelings and overwhelm.

Learning how to tap into your inner calm during pregnancy will serve you well during labor. Mindfulness has been shown to improve one's perception of pain, which has been demonstrated by the popular Lamaze breathing method. Additionally, mindfulness exercises can foster a deep connection between you, your baby, and your body, which can be very empowering. Despite all these benefits, it can be tough to incorporate a new routine into your life and establish a lasting practice. In this chapter, you'll find practical tips to help you embrace and commit to a sustainable lifestyle of open-minded awareness. You'll also find suggestions for how to create a nurturing environment during your mindfulness sessions to make them inviting and comfortable experiences.

Pregnancy Is an Exciting Time

Pregnancy is a unique time of transformation for you and your baby. Witnessing the changes in your body in conjunction with the development of your child will be such a profound and memorable experience, unlike anything else in life. As you settle into the flow of pregnancy and marvel at the wonders of your metamorphosis, you may be overcome by a deepened sense of love and appreciation for your evolving body.

Due to the influx of pregnancy hormones, however, you may also feel a whirlwind of emotions that runs the gamut from excitement and elation to overwhelm, frustration, and fear. Whether this is your first pregnancy or your second, third, or beyond, try to approach each day with patience and grace as you navigate new changes. As you do, be sure to feel the full spectrum of your emotions, as everything you experience is normal.

It is also important to note that every pregnancy journey is unique. If you don't relate to something mentioned in this book, please remember that everyone's experiences will differ, so it does not invalidate your experience. There is no pressure to feel a certain way just because you are pregnant. All experiences and emotions during this time are unique to you, and they are important and valid.

Pregnancy Is Also a Time of Transition and Change

While pregnancy can be a time of excitement and anticipation, it's also a time of transition and change in all aspects of life. The physical changes are obvious, but mental, emotional, and lifestyle shifts are also part of this transformative period. Upon delivering your baby, your role and priorities will move in a different direction, with the responsibility and care of a child bringing a great deal of newness, unpredictability, and pressure. During this transient time, life can feel dramatic and envelop you in a swirl of overwhelm. The exercises in this book will help you feel less consumed by these shifts and more balanced by teaching you awareness, emotional regulation, and a variety of wellness strategies.

Change Can Bring Fear and Worry

Any type of change can breed feelings of angst. So even though you may be excited and happy, moments of worry and fear are normal, too. It's important to create a framework of support for yourself using the tools and tips in this book so you can address your concerns rather than allowing them to fester and become harder to manage. When heightened feelings of stress don't get addressed, they can result in physical symptoms or trigger mood disorders such as anxiety or depression.

According to the March of Dimes, perinatal depression, or depression that occurs during pregnancy and into the first year of having a baby, happens to one in seven women. If you feel overwhelming feelings of sadness or a loss of interest in doing things, please remember that it's okay to ask for help from loved ones or your medical team right away so you can get the necessary support to begin feeling better. Asking for help is a sign of strength, not weakness. Depression is not your fault, nor is it an indication of your ability to be a good parent. You can find resources to help you on page 154.

How Mindfulness Can Help

During this time of creation and transformation, mindfulness can give you an added layer of support to nourish and embolden you. Rather than feeling powerless because you are unsure how to manage your emotions in a healthy way, you can harness the power of awareness to discover new ways of thriving. As your body changes, mindfulness exercises can help you tune in to the areas of your body and mind that need extra attention and love while facilitating connection with your growing baby. During pregnancy, there are also some side effects like stress, worry, fear, anger, and physical discomfort; when these come up, restoration of balance is key. By practicing mindfulness, you'll be able to approach these kinds of situations with intention and meaningful action. In the process, you will expand your consciousness and feel empowered, knowing you have the ability to manage the ups and downs of pregnancy in a way that honors your unique needs.

Getting Comfortable with Your Mind and Body

Cultivating an awareness of both your mind and your body can benefit you during delivery and throughout your pregnancy, especially when your body's changes become more challenging to grasp. Mindfulness practices, such as those rooted in yoga and Qigong, can be intentional and therapeutic, amplifying your physical awareness and reconnecting you to your transforming body. Mindful movement also infuses present-moment connection into exercises aimed at reducing discomfort when your growing body becomes harder to occupy. Other practices, such as meditations and visualizations, enhance feelings of trust, gratitude, and love of yourself and your body. Overall, practicing mindfulness enables you to build a foundation of mental fortitude that will serve you well through the different chapters of pregnancy and delivery.

Connecting to Your Baby

When life gets busy, our connection to ourselves can get muddled. Mindfulness exercises spark an awareness of what's happening within you in real time, such as the growth of your baby. The exercises in this book will give you manageable moments of time to send love, light, and vitality to your developing baby in utero. Techniques like visualization practices can facilitate connection with your child during the first trimester, when they are still too small for you to see or feel any differences. As you start to see growth and feel movement, the practices will continue to build your bond as you talk to your child, write letters to them, and envision delivering your baby and holding them in your arms.

Managing Stress, Worry, and Fear

Whether this is your first pregnancy or fifth, it can feel stressful and scary to create and birth a child, as each experience is unique and comes with its own challenges. There may be times when fear and worry seem to take over because of a medical complication, uneasiness with labor and delivery, or nervousness about becoming a parent. All of these misgivings are common and reasonable. Left unchecked, however, stress can manifest into anxiety, and both can trigger physical symptoms like headaches, tension, fatigue, trouble sleeping, and digestive issues. In pregnancy, high levels of stress and anxiety can also lead to complications during gestation and birth. Fortunately, mindfulness is a very powerful tool that can move you from a heightened state of stress into a calmer, healthier frame of mind.

Relieving Physical Discomfort

As mindfulness exercises spark awareness of your current state of being, they can guide you toward the appropriate self-care for relief. For example, mindfulness exercises such as deep breathing techniques and body scans ease muscle tension and promote overall relaxation of the body. Prenatal exercises offer alternative ways to be mindful while strengthening the body and preparing for the demands of childbirth. Mindful movements like yoga and Qigong improve balance and flexibility while relieving pregnancy symptoms like back pain. As you progress into the second and third trimesters, you may find it difficult to maintain the exercise regimen you used to have. Mindfulness reframes your perception of discomfort and helps you embrace your transformation with a renewed sense of ease and acceptance.

Feeling Empowered

Learning strategies to mitigate stress and fear during your pregnancy journey can be very empowering. Oftentimes, the process of growing a baby can feel like an experience that is happening to us but is out of our hands. Using mindfulness techniques to manage the swell of changes, side effects, and emotions can give you the confidence to navigate your pregnancy in a way that honors your needs. There may be times when you feel intimidated by the mindfulness exercises that push you out of your comfort zone. In those moments, dare to persevere and be vulnerable so you can build your courage and resilience and feel empowered to take on other challenges, like giving birth.

Mindfulness Is Beneficial for Your Baby, Too

One factor dictating a healthy pregnancy is the overall environment in which your baby is growing. Studies have shown that practicing mindfulness during pregnancy can have beneficial effects on the length of time your baby stays in utero, which positively impacts a child's physical and neurological development. Cultivating calm in your life manages your stress levels; it also envelops your child in a nurturing environment that promotes sustained growth.

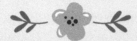

HOW WILL I KNOW IF MY PRACTICE IS HELPING?

As you learn about the many physical, mental, and emotional benefits of practicing mindfulness, I hope you're encouraged to explore and incorporate it into your life. But how will you know that your time and efforts are actually making a difference? There are both immediate and long-term benefits of practicing mindfulness. For example, if you're stressed, by employing a breathing exercise, you can feel the effects immediately, because slowing down your breath sends a signal to your brain that you are moving toward a state of relaxation.

Mindfulness studies conducted on both pregnant women and the general population have demonstrated the following benefits:

Reduced:

+ stress
+ worry
+ anxiety
+ rumination
+ fear
+ reactivity

Increased:

+ calm
+ focus
+ productivity
+ presence
+ tolerance
+ patience
+ trust
+ self-compassion
+ empathy
+ appreciation
+ joy

Although short-term benefits of mindfulness can be realized, such as feeling present and reducing stress in the moment, lasting benefits are dependent on consistent practice.

How to Develop a Sustainable Mindfulness Practice

The habits you develop during your pregnancy inform the person that you want to be during this journey and the person you commit to being as you transition into parenthood. Life can get turned upside-down once you have a newborn. Even your most tried-and-true routines can get tossed out the window because so much of your time is now dedicated to caring for a new life. If you establish a consistent mindfulness practice prior to childbirth, there's a greater chance that awareness will continue to be a part of your daily routine going forward, even if it looks different. By taking care to develop this practice authentically, you can set yourself up for a lifetime of awareness, calm, appreciation, ease, and self-love. The following are some tips to make this new routine accessible and sustainable throughout pregnancy and beyond.

Commit to Five Minutes Per Day

When establishing any new routine, the key to success is your approach. Habits are decisions and actions that are made daily and automatically, sometimes with little conscious thought. Up to 45 percent of what we do daily is habitual action! The goal is to establish your mindfulness practice as one of those daily habits that becomes close to automatic and gets weaved into your identity.

One way to ensure success is to make this new routine easy and approachable. This is where the five-minute time length comes into play. Five minutes is an easy ask because you can squeeze it into any part of your day without it greatly upending your schedule. It is a small commitment with huge rewards and benefits for your wellness.

Stick with It

To make a new habit stick, it's important to understand the framework for successfully establishing a new routine into your life. According to author James Clear, a habit can be broken down into the following loop: cue - craving - response - reward. For those reading this book, the cue is that you are entering a new season of life. The craving, perhaps, is your desire to elevate your wellness during pregnancy and feel more calm, balanced, happy, and connected to your baby. Your response will be your engagement with the exercises in this book on a daily basis. The reward? With each exercise that you complete, you'll begin to feel greater peace, presence, and positivity.

Like with any new habit, you may not feel broad relief immediately. Awareness is a constant feedback loop. When you start to become aware of yourself and your needs, you can then address them using the self-care strategies in this book, which satisfies your craving for restoration. Once you experience this nourishment, you cultivate your ability to be aware and begin to do it more often and over time, even automatically. Showing up for yourself every day and doing these quick exercises sets the foundation for you to access a constant flow of awareness and nourishment.

Find a Quiet Space

It is highly recommended that you begin practicing mindfulness and meditation in a quiet and comfortable space without distractions. Over time, the goal is to practice mindfulness anywhere and anytime once you have strengthened the pathway in your brain to access calm. Until you are at that point, prioritize a quiet location for your daily exercise. Should noises occur during your exercise, gently acknowledge the distraction without judgment and return to your point of focus. You'll learn more about how to deal with distractions later in the book.

Set an Intention

Think of an intention as a road map that guides you along your journey. When you set an intention, you are activating a part of your heart and mind, making them more receptive and aware of the feelings you want to embody in that moment. For example, when you approach your mindfulness practice each day, you can begin by asking yourself, "How do I want to show up for myself today and during this practice?" This question will give you the pause to recognize and dissect how you are currently feeling, and from there you can investigate how you might want to feel differently after the mindfulness exercise.

Try New Practices

Every day is different. With the added layer of hormonal changes during pregnancy, every *minute* can feel different! In order to thrive during pregnancy rather than just survive through it, one key is to tailor your self-care based on how you feel in that moment. Many of the topics and tools included in this book can help you address the wide range of moods and physical symptoms you'll experience throughout your pregnancy journey.

In considering how you feel, challenge yourself to try the various types of exercises highlighted in this book—breathing techniques, visualizations, journaling prompts, gentle movement, meditations, and more. As you try them, you'll see what resonates with you and what might not. Remember that what may not work for you one day may suddenly be really helpful another day, as we are constantly evolving. Allow yourself to stay open to experimentation and the possibilities of growth it may bring.

Stay Open, Aware, and Judgment-Free

A key component of mindfulness is maintaining a judgment-free attitude as you step into any type of awareness exercise. As you open yourself up to experiencing the present, you gain the freedom to authentically explore your inner self without bias or negativity clouding the moment. When you surrender fully to the present, you can transcend into an expansive world of possibility. You might otherwise have suppressed this opportunity because of fear, lack of time, or an inability to access this space. Looking at the present moment nonjudgmentally releases you from the weight of expectations and reframes your approach to focus entirely on yourself and your pregnancy journey.

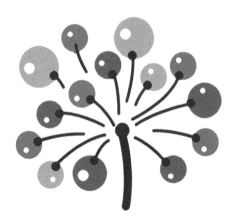

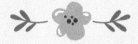

CREATE A NURTURING ENVIRONMENT

Mindfulness is advantageous because you can perform your practice anywhere, anytime, and with little or no special equipment or tools and still experience the many benefits of anchoring to the present moment. Most of the exercises in this book only require a pen, journal, and a timer if desired. If you need to stick to five minutes, set your timer for all the exercises so you can be present in the moment instead of checking your clock.

If you want your daily 5-minute mindfulness sessions to be a more nurturing and peaceful ritual, however, there are some tools that can enhance the experience and even make you feel more inclined to practice. Some of the equipment listed here can make you more comfortable while you practice, especially as you progress into the second and third trimester and require more physical support.

Journal – You can use a notebook, computer, phone, or voice recording program for answering the journaling prompts in this book. Journaling is a great opportunity to allow your thoughts to flow out naturally, unveiling subconscious thinking.

Cushions – Though you can also use a thick pillow, a zafu is a cushion for meditating that encourages your pelvis to tilt forward, your hips to open up, and your back to be supported. This posture support can make your sitting exercises more comfortable and allow you to sit for longer periods if you choose. If you are in a reclined position for an exercise, you can place a bolster or rolled towel under your knees to maintain the natural curvature of your spine. As you enter the third trimester and need more physical support when seated or lying down, feel free to use a full-body pregnancy pillow if you have one.

Candles or essential oils – Candles are a useful addition for ambiance. However, the real benefit of using candles with a scent or essential oils is that using the same scent whenever you practice mindfulness can create an association in your mind, connecting the smell to a state of serenity.

Eye mask – If you find it difficult to keep your eyes closed or find the light distracting even when your eyes are closed, try using an eye mask. The pressure also activates your relaxation response, making you feel calmer.

Blankets – Hormonal changes can create fluctuations in your temperature sensitivity, so blankets can be handy. Weighted blankets can also provide physical comfort when you experience anxiety.

Music – For gentle movement exercises, journaling, or even some meditations, instrumental or meditation background music may help set the mood for you. Much like the use of scents in your practice, you can also create an association with music to the feeling of calm. When it is time to give birth, enlisting the scent and the music can set a tone of serenity during delivery.

Key Takeaways

As we've explored, establishing a consistent mindfulness practice during pregnancy has a multitude of benefits for both you and your baby. Following are some key points to remember on the positive impacts of mindfulness on your pregnancy journey as well as best practices for execution:

✦ During this time of transformation, mindfulness exercises can help you tune in to the areas of yourself that need extra attention and love and facilitate connection with your growing baby.

✦ Mindfulness helps reduce stress and anxiety, resulting in positive effects on your well-being and the development of your baby in utero.

✦ Other benefits of a consistent mindfulness practice include a reduction in overwhelm, fear, reactivity, and the perception of pain, as well as an increase in calm, focus, productivity, patience, trust, tolerance, compassion, gratitude, and joy.

✦ Every pregnancy is unique. Your personal experience, and all your emotions and experiences, are valid and important to honor.

✦ To create a successful routine, approach mindfulness practices using the cue-craving-response-reward framework (page 29), stick to five minutes a day to start, and tie your new habit to an existing ritual, like a bedtime routine or a lunchtime break.

✦ To create a mindfulness practice, all you really need is a quiet space and a nonjudgmental and flexible approach. However, there are some tools, like a journal, scents, music, and pillows, that can enhance your overall experience by physically supporting you and deepening your exploration and connection to calm.

PART TWO

5-Minute Practices

Pregnancy is an exhilarating time of transformation, peppered with an array of emotions from one end of the spectrum to the other. You can empower yourself with strategies and tools to help you manage both the negative and positive emotions that come with bringing a life into this world, using the gift of mindfulness. As you've read, incorporating mindfulness into one's life has many benefits, especially during extraordinary periods of life like pregnancy. Infusing awareness into this time of life can help you become comfortable with your changing body and overworked mind, as well as consciously connect with your baby, manage stress, navigate difficult emotions, relieve physical discomfort, feel emboldened, and nourish your spirit.

The best part is that you will learn realistic and manageable tips on how to build a sustainable mindfulness practice throughout your pregnancy. These approachable recommendations will also help you through the start of your parenting journey, when feeling overwhelmed can prove a daily occurrence. By embracing these short but effective practices, you'll be on your way to building a lasting commitment to a mindful lifestyle.

CHAPTER 3

Calm Your Mind

In this chapter, you will begin your exploration of awareness and apply it to your unique needs. Throughout this special time of development for you and your baby, you will encounter an array of experiences that evoke emotions, both welcome and challenging. The exercises in this chapter will provide you with priceless opportunities to develop your moment-to-moment presence while calming your mind. Specifically, you will learn some basic breathing techniques to ground you to the present and promote relaxation. From this place of calm, you'll uncover the power of responding to life from a place of clarity. You'll also explore some meditations that teach you how to handle thoughts and utilize scents and a mantra. Mixed in are practices that invite you to look inward and reflect upon the present moment, your feelings, your intentions, and your journey thus far. By the end of this chapter, you will have a working knowledge of how to employ mindfulness strategies to uplift your daily life and enhance your overall pregnancy journey.

JOURNAL:

Commitment to Myself

When setting out on any type of exploration, it's always best to have a plan for your course of action or an idea for where you want to go. The same logic applies to one's exploration of oneself and of the present moment. In this journal exercise, you will examine your expectations of your mindfulness practice and its relation to your pregnancy. Part of awareness is recognizing that you have certain ideas so you can challenge their validity to ensure that you are honoring your needs. You will also set an intention, or road map, of commitment to your personal expansion and awakening whenever you do a mindfulness exercise.

1. How are you feeling at this moment about your pregnancy? What do you need to acknowledge about yourself and your current thoughts and feelings?

2. What expectations do you have for your mindfulness practice? What expectations do you have about your pregnancy? Of these, where do you think you can incorporate flexibility when things don't go as planned?

3. What is your overall intention with mindfulness? Write a sentence or two to define your commitment to yourself.

Square Breathing

Breathing strategies are useful calming techniques because you can do them anywhere and at any time–there's no need to close your eyes, be in a quiet space, or use any props. Utilizing a breathing exercise before going into a stressful situation, or even during a stressful moment, can help you minimize your reaction in the heat of the moment. This breathing technique is so effective that it's taught in police departments and the military. The 4-count pattern in this exercise creates a square. You can picture a square in your mind as you breathe if it helps you stay present.

1. Breathe in through your nose for a count of 4 seconds. Notice how the breath is slowly entering your body.

2. Hold your breath for a count of 4 seconds.

3. Breathe out through your nose for a count of 4 seconds. Notice the breath moving out of your body.

4. Hold your breath for a count of 4 seconds.

5. Repeat this pattern as many times as it takes you to feel calmer and better equipped to handle your situation.

MEDITATION:
Thoughts Happen

With so much going on in our lives, it can feel impossible to turn off our thoughts so we can meditate. Rather than trying to shut your mind off completely, think of your meditation as an exercise in acknowledging your thoughts without judgment and just letting them go. Reframing meditation in this manner reminds you that you are not your thoughts and prevents you from engaging with them. Instead, consider yourself the observer of your thoughts. When you do so, it can feel easier to let them go.

1. Sit or lie down. Close your eyes.
2. Ground into the present by taking 2 deep breaths through your nose.
3. Witness your breath as it moves in and out of your body.
4. When a thought pops up in your mind, gently acknowledge the thought by saying in your head, "Thoughts happen." Try not to judge yourself or the thought.
5. Release the thought by visualizing it going away, such as putting it on a cloud and pushing it away. Use any visualization that works for you.
6. Resume taking deep breaths and witnessing your breath.
7. If thoughts arise again, follow steps 4 through 6 each time.
8. When the timer ends, open your eyes.

Seated Forward Bend

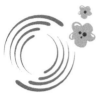

Amid the joys of pregnancy, this experience can also come with discomfort. The movement exercises in this book will channel awareness of your body to strengthen the vital connection of your mind to your physical being. In this seated exercise, you will connect to your lower back and the backs of your legs as you release and stretch them.

1. Sit with your legs out in front of you, slight bend in the knees. Spread your legs if you need room for your growing belly.

2. Before bending forward, take a deep breath through your nose.

3. Keeping your back as straight as possible, bend at the hips, reaching your hands toward your toes.

4. As you reach forward, gently exhale from your mouth. With every breath, feel yourself relax more deeply into this position.

5. Only reach as far as is comfortable. Stop if you feel pain.

6. If you can bend forward a bit more, continue to reach toward your toes while gently breathing.

7. If needed, you can sit up for a break or to reset. Then repeat steps 2 through 4.

8. Remain in your seated forward bend while breathing deeply through your nose until your timer ends.

JOURNAL:
Digging Deep

To know when we need to care for ourselves, we need to recognize how we are feeling in the moment. Unfortunately, the busyness of life often dulls our connection to our physical body and emotional state. Then there are times when we purposefully avoid tuning in to ourselves because we're afraid of confronting our truths. Take this time to check in on how you are feeling today. This is a great way to show up for yourself and make space for whatever wants to come to the surface. Choose one or more of the following prompts to answer in your journal.

1. How are you feeling right now? If you feel worried, stressed, or anxious, try to uncover the reasons why you feel this way. Did something happen to trigger you?

2. Honor your emotions, whether they are positive or not, by acknowledging, allowing, and validating them. With this knowledge, brainstorm and write about ways that you can avoid or manage triggering situations that lead to negative emotions in the future.

3. How can you be true to yourself? Consider your thoughts, emotions, and desires.

MEDITATION:

Aromatherapy

Aromatherapy is the use of scents in therapeutic practices. You can use scents from essential oils, candles, or perfumes to enhance your connection to calm. Find a scent that is pleasing to you and experiment throughout your pregnancy. It is important to know, however, that some essential oils are not safe for use during pregnancy. Calming oils that are safe to use after the first trimester with the approval of your healthcare provider include lavender, chamomile, bergamot, and ylang-ylang. Ideally, use one scent consistently during your daily mindfulness practice to connect that scent to a feeling of calm. Use that scent during delivery to provide increased tranquility.

1. Light a candle. If using an essential oil, place a drop of oil on a tissue, or on the insides of your wrists and rub together.

2. Sit or lie down. Close your eyes.

3. Slowly inhale and breathe in the scent. If you are using an essential oil, you may need to bring the scent closer to your nose.

4. Slowly exhale through your nose.

5. Repeat step 3 while saying in your mind, "I am calm." Then exhale slowly.

6. Continue breathing through your nose, periodically bringing the scent up to your nose as you inhale and saying the phrase "I am calm."

7. When the timer ends, gently open your eyes.

BREATHWORK:
Deep Belly Breath

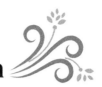

How often do you notice how you are breathing? Shallow breaths or holding our breath can actually trigger a stress response. Shorter breaths also rob us of potential energy because we aren't getting enough oxygen into our system, which helps with energy levels. When we breathe from our diaphragm, the muscle at the base of the lungs, we have a greater capacity to inhale than by breathing from our chest. Diaphragmatic breathing, however, may feel harder to do as your belly grows. In this exercise, do the best you can without straining.

1. Lie down using props such as pillows or rolled blankets for comfort.

2. Place one hand on your belly and the other hand on your chest to remind yourself where to originate your breath.

3. Inhale, beginning your breath from your belly and pushing your belly outward. Imagine filling your belly with air as it expands.

4. Exhale, releasing the air through your nose, and witness your belly deflating. Notice your hand moving down.

5. Continue this process of deep breathing. Feel relaxation washing over you. With each breath, you are taking in more oxygen and releasing carbon dioxide, promoting equilibrium and serenity.

6. When the timer ends, gently open your eyes.

My Choice

Do you ever feel like your emotions and thoughts are out of your control, especially during pregnancy? If so, remember that you have the power to adjust your relationship to your thoughts. Thoughts come and go, and you can choose to hold on to them or let them go. It is also in your power to choose what you think afterward. By adjusting your relationship with your thoughts, you can shift your mindset. You can start just by choosing the words you use to describe how you feel. Follow the prompts below to see how you can choose your attitude with intention.

1. Write down the statement "It is my choice to feel_____" several times. Fill in the blanks with various emotions you want to embody, such as calm, brave, beautiful, confident, limitless, etc.

2. During this time of reflection, observe your thoughts. If a difficult thought pops up, try to follow it with an alternate thought that offers love, compassion, support, or encouragement. How did it feel to stop a negative process and choose a more positive replacement idea instead?

MEDITATION:
Be Here Now

A mantra is a vehicle for the mind to stay grounded to the present moment. It can be a word, phrase, sound, or even words in another language. When using a mantra, repeat it softly in the back of your mind, allowing it to be gentle in its presence, almost like a song you keep singing in your mind. Mantras can also be used outside of meditation, whenever you need words of encouragement or a reminder to stay focused.

1. Find a comfortable seated or reclined position and close your eyes.

2. Tap into the present by taking 2 deep breaths through your nose.

3. Notice your breath moving in and out of your body. Allow the outside world to fade away with each deep breath.

4. On your next breath, gently say the words "Be here now" in your mind as you inhale. Then gently exhale.

5. Continue repeating this mantra as you breathe.

6. If you find your mind wandering, acknowledge the distracted thought without judgment and use a visualization for releasing the thought (see page 41, step 5). Then say your mantra to help you anchor yourself back to the present moment.

7. When your timer ends, gently open your eyes.

Vagus Nerve

The vagus nerve goes from your belly up to your face, sending sensory information to your brain. It helps with immunity and inflammation and releases hormones that aid in relaxation. One way to stimulate your vagus nerve is to use an eye pillow when sleeping, but in this exercise, you'll learn how to stimulate your vagus nerve by applying light pressure around your eyes. You can also pair this with an essential oil placed on your wrists (see page 44 for safe, calming oils for pregnancy). This exercise is easy to do anywhere and anytime you need to access calm.

1. Rub your palms together gently, creating a little heat.

2. After a few seconds, close your eyes and lightly place your warmed palms over your eye area.

3. Take a few deep breaths while repeating the mantra "I am giving myself a gift of peace" in your mind.

4. Notice the warmth of your hands. Imagine the heat moving from your hands to your eyes and a soothing energy flowing into your being, restoring balance and vitality.

5. If the heat dissipates, rub your hands together again and replace them gently over your eyes. Breathe deeply and repeat your mantra.

6. When your timer ends, softly remove your hands from your eyes.

Ocean Breath

Taking a deep breath in the midst of chaos is like hitting the pause button on life. In doing so, you honor your need for restoration. We know that breathing techniques move us into a state of calm and presence, but the accompanying pause gives us clarity by providing the space to view our situation with perspective. By centering yourself with your breath, you can then proceed peacefully with purpose, even in overwhelming situations. Use this technique anytime you feel anxious, such as at a doctor's appointment.

1. Take a slow, deep breath in through your nose, taking in only as much air as feels comfortable.

2. Without pausing, flow your inhale directly into a slow exhale out of your nose.

3. When you reach the end of your exhale, flow directly into your next inhale.

4. Continue to flow your inhale and exhale directly into one another without pausing.

5. With each breath, allow yourself to release stress and invite relaxation within.

6. If you need a visual to help you stay grounded, imagine the ocean waves flowing into the shore and immediately retreating back out in a continuous fashion.

Challenge Accepted

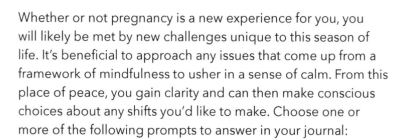

Whether or not pregnancy is a new experience for you, you will likely be met by new challenges unique to this season of life. It's beneficial to approach any issues that come up from a framework of mindfulness to usher in a sense of calm. From this place of peace, you gain clarity and can then make conscious choices about any shifts you'd like to make. Choose one or more of the following prompts to answer in your journal:

1. Reflect on a time you came upon an obstacle. This can be from before or during your pregnancy. How did you react or respond? Why do you think you approached your situation this way?

2. When you encounter a challenge, do you allow yourself to acknowledge the difficulties of the situation and be vulnerable? This vulnerability can include asking for help, having a good cry, or doing anything else that honors your feelings. Are there ways that you can lean into these moments and grow from them?

3. Do you notice any patterns in how you respond to challenging times? Can you think of alternate, more helpful ways to respond to similar scenarios in the future?

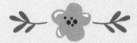

INTENTIONAL TRANSITIONS

The ceremony you hold around your meditation, visualization, movement, or breathwork exercise matters just as much as the heart of the practice. This means taking your time, especially not to rush into your mindfulness session or rush out of it; this becomes particularly important if you are lying down and are further along in your pregnancy. Before beginning, give yourself a moment to just breathe with your eyes open. Let a few audible sighs out of your mouth. This signals, "I'm here. I made it. These next five minutes are just for me to refresh and nourish myself."

When you finish an exercise, give yourself another moment to let stillness settle within you. Before getting up, wiggle your fingers and toes to reconnect to your body. If you're lying down, maybe turn on your side and prop yourself up with your hands to move gently into a seated position and then stand. By moving slowly and intentionally, you hold on to the serenity that you just cultivated.

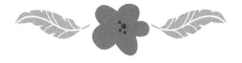

CHAPTER 4

Empower Your Body

This chapter is dedicated to honoring your magnificent body for all it is masterfully taking on during your pregnancy journey. During this transformative period, it can be easy to fall into self-judgment and comparisons to others, especially in a digital age that idealizes certain ways of looking and feeling. Remember, you are beautiful and capable. To strengthen this belief, the exercises in this chapter will focus on showing yourself kindness and compassion and honoring your individuality, which can lead to improvements in confidence and overall well-being.

The strategies in this chapter will also enhance your mind-body connection, reconcile your views, and amplify your acceptance of your body's changes. Mindfulness tools can remind you to pay attention and nurture your body as a form of self-love, self-care, and restoration. Also included are practices that will aid in the management of discomfort and pain associated with pregnancy and childbirth. By tuning in to your body mindfully on a daily basis, you give yourself the opportunity to check in, be present in your own skin, and address your ever-changing needs.

Caring for My Pregnant Self

During this unique time in your life, you will witness many physical changes to your body, including some that will astonish you. As you progress through pregnancy, these changes will also require shifts in how you care for yourself. The following prompts are designed to activate your awareness of your physical and mental state, guiding you on a path toward nourishment. Reflect and respond to the following prompts in your journal:

1. Pay attention to how your body feels throughout each week of your pregnancy. Write down symptoms, physical changes, energy levels, current emotions, and anything else that feels relevant to this stage of your experience.

2. Based on your pregnancy thus far, come up with a list of ways to care for yourself and address any issues you are experiencing. For example, if you have swollen feet, give yourself Epsom salt foot soaks and wear compression socks. Once you're in the midst of discomfort, it can be hard to remember all the ways that you can alleviate your symptoms. You may find that you resort to the same approaches repeatedly. Having a list, however, provides options to turn to. This list is also helpful to share with anyone in your support system so they can feel empowered to help you.

Cat-Cow Pose

The added weight in front of your body that comes with a growing baby causes major strain on the back and hips. To counter this strain, cat-cow is great for stretching the back and maintaining a flexible spine. With all moves in this book, make each movement mindful by focusing on the connection of your breath with your body, noticing how each pose feels. A modification to this pose is to sit in a chair.

1. Get on all fours with your palms on the ground, keeping your hands underneath your shoulders, knees under your hips. Alternately, sit in a chair.

2. Throughout this exercise, exhale from your mouth as you move into each position.

3. To move into cow pose, exhale and let your belly drop, slightly arching your back while gently lifting your tailbone and your head and chin up toward the sky. Hold for a few deep breaths. If seated, move your shoulders and head back as your belly pushes forward, creating an arch in your back while in your seated position.

4. Move into cat pose by exhaling through your mouth, tucking your chin to your chest, squeezing your abdominals inward, and rounding your back up toward the sky (or the back of the chair). Feel for a gentle stretch between your shoulder blades. Hold for a few deep breaths.

5. Repeat steps 3 and 4 as time permits.

Trust My Body

If this is your first pregnancy or if you are experiencing any complications, it can be hard to trust your body. It can be even harder to believe in your body if you had a difficult time getting pregnant. The gestational process is an education in letting go and relying on trust, courage, and flexibility. This meditation will help you channel confidence in yourself and ignite your inner radiance.

1. Find a comfortable seated or reclined position and close your eyes.

2. Take 2 deep breaths through your nose. Witness the calm that washes over you with each breath.

3. Allow your breath to return to a comfortable pace.

4. In your mind, say the following mantra: "With each breath, I cultivate trust in myself, my body, and my capacity for radiant health."

5. With each inhale and exhale, repeat this mantra to yourself. Feel the words taking root within you with every inhale.

6. If you feel your mind wandering, acknowledge the thoughts without judgment and send them out of your mind. Know that you can return to them once you are done prioritizing your well-being.

7. When the timer ends, gently open your eyes.

Comparison Is the Thief of Joy

It's human nature to use other people as a benchmark for success. In this digital age, however, it's a lot easier to compare ourselves to many unrealistic versions of what it means to be a pregnant person. Oftentimes, when we see an image of what the "perfect" pregnancy should look and be like, it can make our own experience and emotions here in the real world feel invalid. When you see other representations of pregnancy, do your best not to compare or let your joy turn into feelings of jealousy, unworthiness, or frustration. To help you grapple with these feelings, choose one or both of the following prompts to answer in your journal:

1. List the things you love about yourself. Add to this list throughout your pregnancy journey. When you feel insecure or your spirits are low, review this list to remind yourself of your unique, remarkable qualities.

2. What insecurities have you had in the past that you've overcome? How were you able to do this? Can you apply the same methods to any pregnancy insecurities?

Permission to Rest

As time goes on, it can become harder to feel comfortable and rest in your own body due to the physical and hormonal changes you experience. In this meditation, you'll give yourself permission to rest when you feel like you are pushing yourself too hard to take care of tasks or maintain your pre-pregnancy activities. This is your reminder that it's okay to take a "time-in," because your body is working hard to create a life.

1. Lie in bed. Close your eyes.

2. Breathe deeply as you say the mantra "I welcome rest into my being" in your mind.

3. Breathe in and out deeply through your nose and note 30.

4. Breathe deeply and note 29.

5. Continue to count down. With each counted breath, welcome rest into every part of your body and feel yourself softening into the bed beneath you.

6. When you get down to 1, take a deep breath. Repeat your mantra.

7. Lie restfully, witnessing how your body feels while accepting rest. Breathe deeply into this state of relaxation, repeating your mantra.

8. When your timer ends, gently open your eyes.

MOVEMENT:
Wide Child's Pose

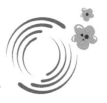

This yoga pose is a restorative grounding pose that opens your hips and lengthens your spine. Doing a wide version of child's pose gives space for your growing belly, while also widening your hips, preparing you for childbirth. A cushion or yoga block is helpful if you can't touch your forehead to the ground.

1. Sit with your legs folded underneath you, legs open wide, calves touching the ground, arms raised overhead.

2. With your back straight, slowly fold forward from the hips, exhaling through your mouth until your head lands on the ground or a supportive device, and your outstretched arms fall on either side of your head. Allow your forehead to touch the ground or device, or turn your head to the side.

3. Adjust as needed, spreading your knees out more to the sides to make room for your belly and moving your shoulders away from your ears.

4. Breathe slowly and deeply in this position. With each breath, feel your body relaxing while welcoming expansion and restoration. Only stretch as far as is comfortable.

5. If needed, you can sit up for a break or to reset. Then repeat steps 2 through 4.

6. End the pose by sitting up slowly, using your hands to help you up if needed.

Body Breath

Your breath is a powerful tool that can move you into a state of calm. You can also direct your breath to specific spots along your body to facilitate targeted relaxation or infuse energy into that space. In this exercise, your hands provide extra guidance for your breath. It can be especially useful for people new to breathing techniques to have a physical cue for where to focus their breath and attention.

1. Sit or lie down. Close your eyes.
2. Take 2 deep breaths through your nose.
3. Allow your breath to return to a comfortable pace.
4. Place both hands over your heart or the center of your chest.
5. On your next breath, try to direct the breath to where you feel your hands on your body. Alternatively, just feel that spot where your hands are placed, noticing movement with each breath.
6. Take 3 deep breaths into this space.
7. Repeat steps 5 and 6, moving your hands to the following places:
    a. Forehead or the space between your eyebrows
    b. Throat
    c. Belly
8. End with 2 deep breaths in through your nose and out through your mouth.
9. When the timer ends, gently open your eyes.

A Shout-Out to Myself

Gratitude is a powerful tool that can move a person from a negative frame of mind to a more appreciative and positive mindset. We give thanks to others, but how often do we shower ourselves with love and appreciation? It's time! Tune in to all the remarkable changes your body has gone through and that will continue to occur. The significance of this transformation is immense. Writing a letter to yourself is a cathartic exercise that will open your eyes to your strength and courage. Consider adding this letter to your delivery bag so you can give yourself a boost of love, support, and empowerment before giving birth.

1. Before you put pen to paper, take some time to sit and reflect on all that your body has done for you so far. You can even think about times prior to pregnancy.

2. Now think about all the things that your body will continue to do throughout your pregnancy, during labor and delivery, and then afterward to repair itself and care for your newborn.

3. Write a letter of acknowledgment and appreciation for your body. Consider this your personal love letter to yourself.

MEDITATION:
I Am Creating Life

Let's be clear—you are a *champion* for all the profound work you are doing in creating a life! It can be hard to comprehend the magnitude of what's happening during the first trimester, when you may not even feel like you are pregnant. In this meditation, you'll remind yourself that you are phenomenal for creating a life. Whenever you feel down, uplift yourself by repeating the following mantra as you take slow, deep breaths. Allow these words to reconnect you to your inner power and light.

1. Find a comfortable seated or reclined position and close your eyes.

2. Settle into the present moment by witnessing your slow, deep breaths.

3. Place your hands on your belly and observe your belly rising and falling with each breath.

4. On every inhale, gently repeat this mantra in your mind: "I am creating a life within me." Then slowly exhale out through your nose.

5. Continue repeating this mantra to yourself and feel the words embedding within your heart and mind. With every breath, connect to your inner light and strength. Recognize a frequency of radiance, vitality, and power.

6. When your timer ends, gently open your eyes.

JOURNAL:

Body Acceptance

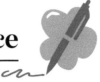

As your body changes, it may not look or feel the way you want. When expectations clash with reality, it can create turbulent emotions. While you don't always have to feel positive about your pregnancy transformation, you can learn to accept what is happening in a mindful way and honor your feelings. Unlike body positivity, body acceptance gives you room to love your pregnant body and be okay with feeling bothered by the weight gain, stretch marks, and/or your overall appearance. Choose one or more prompts to answer in your journal:

1. How are you coping with your transformation? Write down how you are feeling about the changes to your body.

2. Address any unrealistic expectations you have for your pregnancy body and explore how you can dismantle these beliefs. Challenge negative thinking by offering a counterargument for each expectation you list.

3. Do you have any fears about future body changes? Try writing a coping strategy next to each fear for when this concern bubbles up in the future.

4. Write some affirming statements about your pregnancy body to use on the days you're feeling down about your appearance and need a shift in perspective.

MEDITATION:
Body Scan

This exercise identifies areas of stress, and it relaxes and grounds the body. A body scan can be done as a meditation or as a standalone practice, such as when you first wake up, while working, at doctor's appointments, or at bedtime to establish a connection with your body.

1. Sit or lie down. Close your eyes.

2. Begin by noticing your lower body—feet, ankles, calves, knees, and thighs.

3. Observe any tightness or discomfort.

4. Inhale. Visualize breathing into those areas of tension. Imagine your breath expanding in those areas while saying, "I am present in my body."

5. Exhale and visualize the tension flowing out of your body via your breath.

6. Witness your midsection—glutes, pelvis, belly, chest, and back. Repeat steps 3 through 5.

7. Observe your hands, arms, shoulders, and neck. Repeat steps 3 through 5. Before exhaling, bring your shoulders up to your ears and let them fall away from your ears as you exhale.

8. Witness your head—jaws, the corners of your eyes, and your forehead. Repeat steps 3 through 5. Open your mouth slightly to release any jaw clenching. Use your hand to rub any furrow in your brow. Release any squint in your closed eyes.

9. End by taking 2 deep breaths through your nose, and notice all the spaciousness you have created.

MOVEMENT:

Savasana/Corpse Pose

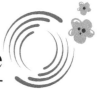

This pose, held at the end of all yoga sessions, may seem like a glorified nap, but it's actually a powerful exercise in resting awareness, where you give yourself permission to surrender to peaceful restoration. Use whatever props you need to fully give in to this moment of renewal—pillows, blankets, eye coverings, etc.

1. Lie down in a comfortable position, using props to enhance relaxation.

2. Close your eyes. Inhale through your nose.

3. Make an audible sigh from your mouth.

4. Return your breath to a soft pace.

5. Scan your body for any areas of tension. Use your breath to soften these spots and exhale the tension.

6. After your body scan, notice your breath. With every inhalation, invite stillness into your being. Feel the unconditional support from the earth beneath you.

7. With every exhale, feel yourself melting further into the ground, relaxing deeper into this position.

8. To end the pose, wiggle your fingers and toes and open your eyes. Gently roll to one side and use your hands to help you sit upright.

9. Close your practice by taking a deep breath. Extend gratitude to yourself for taking time to nourish and restore your body and mind.

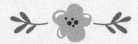

PRIORITIZE YOURSELF

By committing to these daily exercises, you are prioritizing yourself. Self-care is not a luxury, nor is it selfish. Self-care facilitates improvement in your overall well-being.

Take a moment to consider how these practices have worked for you. Have you been able to keep up with a daily routine of doing one 5-minute exercise each day? If not, don't beat yourself up—getting sidetracked happens. Flexibility and grace are essential when establishing a new habit. Your continued effort to cultivate awareness and practice self-care strategies during your pregnancy will serve you well as you transition into parenthood. When life gets more demanding, you will know how to fit in at least five minutes to mother yourself so you can better care for others.

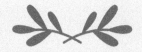

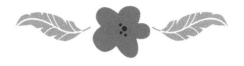

CHAPTER 5

Connect with Your Baby

Sometimes it can feel difficult to establish a connection with your baby during pregnancy, especially during the early stages when you don't look pregnant and can't feel your baby in your belly. In this chapter, you'll find a mix of dynamic and effective strategies to help you cultivate a strong connection with your baby in utero, even though you haven't met yet. You will use the power of your voice and music to forge a meaningful bond with your child, as sound is known to travel into the womb. The journaling exercises in this section will challenge you to look inward and surrender to the beauty of your present-moment experience. The meditations and visualizations will provide opportunities to vividly imagine your baby and your life together. So even though your child is not yet out here in the world with you, you can still build an emotional and conscious connection with them through these practices that will invoke and amplify love and care. In short, this chapter encourages you to transition from thinking of yourself as merely a pregnant person to slowly embracing and practicing the joys of being a parent.

First Ultrasound

The first time you see your baby via ultrasound is a wondrous occasion. Visuals like pictures or live scans can make a pregnancy feel more "real" and abate any trepidations about the viability of the pregnancy and the health of your baby. Keep that special memory of connection with your child alive by writing about your experience in detail using the following prompts. If you have already had this appointment, feel free to either recall your experience or wait until your next scan to complete this writing exercise. At upcoming appointments, try to stay grounded in what is happening while allowing all outside thoughts and worries to flow in and out of your mind without judgment or attachment.

1. Describe the details of the experience—sounds, smells, sights.

2. What thoughts and emotions did you have when you first laid eyes on your baby on the monitor?

3. Did you stay present in that moment? If you feel like there's room for improvement in your awareness, what were the distractions and what are some ways you can be more mindful during future ultrasounds and appointments?

My Growing Baby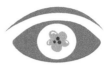

During your first trimester, it can be difficult to grasp the idea of your pregnancy, as you may not look or feel pregnant. That's where this exercise comes in. Any time you want to connect with your baby throughout the early stages of pregnancy, do the following visualization exercise.

1. Find a comfortable seated or reclined position.

2. Close your eyes when you feel ready.

3. Begin to anchor to the moment by witnessing your slow, deep breathing initiated from the belly.

4. Place one or both hands on your belly.

5. With every inhale, allow your belly to expand outward and feel the energy you are creating. By observing your belly's expansion and the energy created in that area, you are connecting with your baby.

6. Repeat the following mantra out loud as often as you like: "I am holding space for you to flourish in my love."

7. Imagine that every breath you take, you are strengthening your connection to your baby.

8. With every rise of your belly, visualize your baby growing from a tiny embryo into a little baby and repeat the mantra for your baby to hear.

9. When your timer ends, gently open your eyes.

AWARENESS EXERCISE:
Cultivating Connections

Have you ever noticed how songs from the past can spark a flood of memories and emotions? This is because of how our brain processes and retains music. Likewise, you can encourage your brain to forge *new* connections of calm with specific songs during your pregnancy.

Pick one song to use during this exercise and feel free to play it softly in the background during your other daily mindfulness practices. It can be instrumental, meditational, or anything soothing to you. Throughout your pregnancy, select other songs to gradually build a small playlist to use during labor and delivery to create a calming atmosphere. When you hear these songs, you'll instantly be transported to your daily moments of peace and happiness.

1. Turn your song on at a soft volume.
2. Sit or lie down and close your eyes.
3. Take slow, intentional breaths.
4. Witness the movement in your torso created by your breath while listening to the music in the background.
5. Softly repeat this mantra: "I am filled with serenity as these sounds float into my being."
6. Feel the calming vibrations of the music with every deep inhale and exhale.
7. Open your eyes when the song ends.

BREATHWORK:

Alternate Nostril Breathing

This breathing technique invokes restoration and relaxation. If you're congested, do this on another day. Even when you're healthy, one nostril might be more open than the other—this is common. Take it slowly and gradually build up your capacity. Stop if you feel light-headed.

1. Sit in a comfortable position with your eyes closed or open with a soft gaze.

2. Bring your right hand up to your nose and bend your index and middle fingers down toward your palm.

3. Place your right thumb over your right nostril, closing off the nasal passage.

4. Inhale slowly and deeply through your left nostril.

5. While still closing off the right nostril with your thumb, exhale slowly through your left nostril.

6. Close your left nostril by pressing down with your ring finger and release your thumb off of your right nostril.

7. Breathe slowly and deeply into your right nostril.

8. Exhale slowly through your right nostril.

9. Witness the movement of the breath through your body. Zero in on the feeling of energy that you are creating through this active breath. Imagine the breath revitalizing you while ushering in tranquility.

10. Repeat steps 3 through 8 for as long as you are able or until your timer ends.

Movement Reflections

The first time you feel your baby moving, write about your experience so you can lock this profound occasion into your memory. Writing in your journal about special times in life gives you the ability to relive those priceless moments anytime you like. It can also help you unearth and examine any emotions intertwined with that situation. When you reread these journal entries in the future, you'll also reconnect to a version of yourself that may be quite different from who you've become.

1. The first time you feel movement in your belly, describe in detail everything in that moment: location, time, sights, smells, your clothing, who was with you, what you were doing, etc.

2. Now, describe what the movement actually felt like to you.

3. Journal about your feelings at that moment. (Remember, being honest in your writing details the full spectrum of your experience versus creating a picture-perfect version that isn't authentic. Even if you feel scared or nervous, share your truth and own your story.)

4. The movements in your belly will change dramatically over time. Use this same journaling exercise to describe your experiences in the future, making note of differences from previous movements.

MOVEMENT:

Bound Angle

In this yoga pose, invite revitalization into your being. It's a great move to do after exercising to stretch and rebalance. As you progress in your pregnancy, this pose can alleviate discomfort in your lower back. It also opens your hips, making it conducive for birth preparation. For extra support, set a folded blanket or towel under your hips.

1. Sit on the ground with a straight spine. Bring the bottoms of your feet together. The closer your feet are to your groin, the deeper the stretch. Adjust the distance to your comfort. Feel for a gentle stretch in your inner thighs and hips, with your knees not rising past your hip level.

2. Wrap your hands around your feet, and use the aid of your elbows to press down on your knees for a deeper stretch if desired.

3. Inhale deeply through your nose.

4. Keeping a straight back, exhale slowly as you bend at your hips toward your feet with your gaze following. Only bend as far as you feel a gentle stretch. Breathe deeply as you hold the pose. Use your exhale to move deeper into the stretch if desired.

5. If needed, you can sit up for a break or to reset. Then repeat steps 2 through 4.

Baby Shushing Breath

Many babies love falling asleep to white noise, as it mimics the sounds in the womb enveloping them in comfort. A crying baby can instantly send parents into a state of stress. By learning this breathing technique now, it will help you in the present, and in the future, it will calm both you and your baby simultaneously.

1. Sit or lie down in a comfortable position with your eyes closed.

2. Take a deep inhale through your nose.

3. When you exhale, breathe out loudly through your mouth making a "shhh" sound. Extend the shhh exhale for as long as you can.

4. As you inhale, tune in to your belly rising up as it fills up with a big breath.

5. As you exhale audibly with a shhh, observe your belly falling down and inward as it releases both air and any tension that you may be holding on to. Use this opportunity as your chance to unwind and let go of stress.

6. Repeat this breath until your timer ends. Gently open your eyes and allow the calm that you cultivated during this practice to serve as the foundation for the rest of your day.

MEDITATION:
Sending Love to My Belly

In this meditation, you will combine a mantra and visualization to connect deeply with your baby.

1. Find a comfortable seated or reclined position. Close your eyes.

2. Anchor to this moment by witnessing your breath as it moves in and out of your body.

3. Place both hands over your womb.

4. Allow your breath to start from your belly, if possible, and mentally observe the rise and fall of your belly with every slow, deep breath.

5. Imagine that your breath is the love and energy you are sending to your baby to help them grow.

6. Take a deep breath, then gently repeat this mantra out loud for your baby to hear: "I am enveloping you in my unconditional love."

7. Allow each breath to come from a place of intention and love, and imagine your breath as the flow of love going into your womb and surrounding your baby.

8. If you feel movement during this meditation, gently move your hands to the place where you feel your baby moving. Focus your breath on the space where your hands are placed and imagine that you are directly connected via that area.

9. Open your eyes when your timer ends.

Chatting with My Baby

Babies start to hear sounds at around the 18th week of pregnancy, and they hear sounds from outside the womb at around 6 to 7 months. In this exercise, build your bond with your baby by talking out loud and sharing any thoughts, feelings, or life experiences.

1. You can do this exercise anywhere you feel comfortable talking out loud. For example, describe the rooms in your home, especially their nursery space, or go for a walk and narrate your experience.

2. As you talk to your baby, try rubbing your belly, either over your clothes or directly on your skin with belly cream or massage oil if desired. By adding physical touch to your baby talk, you can deepen your connection to your child as you incorporate another point of awareness into the moment. Babies also begin to feel when you touch your belly around month 4 of pregnancy and eventually will respond to your touch with movement.

3. While talking to your baby, make the experience more mindful by observing how you feel in the moment and how your baby responds to your voice and touch.

4. Journal about the experience after each time you talk to your baby, or as often as you wish.

A Letter to My Baby

Take a moment to reflect on the magnitude of the pregnancy process and your honest feelings about your pregnancy journey thus far. Then write a letter to your baby, using any or all of the following prompts to spark your authentic flow. If you'd like, you can use one prompt each time for different letters to your child that you can share with them in the future.

1. Describe this journey of cultivating connection with your baby, sharing any highlights or tough moments, along with the ways your bond has developed.

2. Begin your letter with "Before even meeting you, I love you because . . . "

3. Begin with "As a parent, these are my hopes and dreams for you." After listing your personal expectations for them, write an acknowledgment honoring their individuality and their ability to forge their own path, sharing your support for them. (Expectations for our children can be difficult to release as parents, because we want the best for them. It may be helpful to also visualize and acknowledge other paths for them to help open your mind to alternative journeys.)

4. Begin with "I can't wait to be your parent because . . . "

Holding My Baby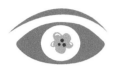

Harnessing the power of imagery can help you navigate tough days during pregnancy and pivot toward positivity and hopefulness. The key to visualization is using the five senses as much as possible when picturing a moment; this will make it feel real in your mind. Implement this visualization when you feel disconnected from the ultimate goal of having a baby and need a vivid reminder.

1. Find a comfortable seated or reclined position. Close your eyes.

2. Place both hands on your belly.

3. Take 2 deep breaths.

4. Picture yourself sitting at home with your baby. In your mind, look around and observe everything about this moment—sights, sounds, smells, textures, temperature. What are you wearing? How do you feel? Envision yourself however you like. You can be exhausted, glowing, uncomfortable, joyful, etc.

5. Look down in your arms and see the beautiful baby you are holding. How do you feel when you look at your child?

6. Witness the smile that spreads across your face. Feel the intensity of love as you lock eyes with your baby. With every breath, allow these feelings to take root within.

7. When your timer ends, allow your visualization to gently fade away for now. Gently open your eyes.

8. Write down some highlights of your visualization.

Birthing Affirmations

During the birth of your child, it can greatly help to use certain phrases or affirmations to keep you confident, empowered, calm, and strong during the last part of your pregnancy. Using the following prompts, create simple sentences you can say to yourself or have your partner or birthing coach say to you during labor and delivery or as you prepare for your C-section. Print out a list for your support team, and consider having them written on paper for you to see in the room as visual reminders.

1. Think about the birth of your child and the parts of the process that worry or scare you the most. What words of encouragement do you want to hear to offset those concerns?

2. Labor and delivery can be a long and taxing process, and a C-section may sound daunting, but remember that you are a phenomenal being. What are some affirmations you'd like to remember during that time? Affirmations are "I am" statements that act as reminders of how you see yourself or how you ideally want to be. Examples: "I am strong." "I am limitless." "I am courageous." "I am a goddess." "I can do this."

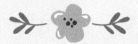

BIRTHING PREP

Cultivating a mindset of calm will serve you well when you get to the point of labor and delivery. To assist in creating an environment of tranquility during the final stage of pregnancy, pack some items in your hospital bag that are geared toward your self-care and creating a peaceful sanctuary:

✦ Essential oils used during your aromatherapy practice (see page 44)

✦ This book

✦ Your journal and a few writing utensils

✦ The letters you wrote to yourself and your baby via the prompts in this book (see page 61 and 77)

✦ The music you used to create your calm connection (see page 70) and a mini speaker

✦ Your birthing affirmations and mantra (see page 75 and 79) on paper

✦ A lacrosse or tennis ball for the partner massage exercise (see page 120)

✦ Other favorite items that promote serenity and wellness

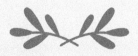

CHAPTER 6

Make Peace with Difficult Emotions

There's an adage that says the only way out of a difficult situation is through it. Facing our fears, worries, doubts, or sadness can feel like an insurmountable task. Wouldn't it just be easier to deal with it later? The problem with repressing feelings, however, is that the heaviness of those emotions still weighs on you, causing a variety of physical and mental repercussions.

The benefit of learning and regularly practicing mindfulness is that it arms you with the tools and support to be vulnerable, face difficult emotions, and come through stronger. With mindfulness as your foundation, you realize you are not identified by your thoughts and feelings, and this realization gives way to an expansive feeling of freedom and peace, leading to a more fulfilled life.

The exercises in this chapter will stop the cycle of any repeating patterns for dealing with hardships that aren't productive or positive. Instead, you will take the bold move to step out of your comfort zone and confront any feelings of sadness, jealousy, shame, self-doubt, frustration, or anger and transcend into courageous expansion, unfettered by the weight of negativity.

Emotional Awareness

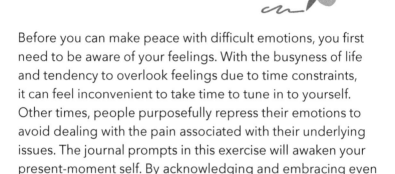

Before you can make peace with difficult emotions, you first need to be aware of your feelings. With the busyness of life and tendency to overlook feelings due to time constraints, it can feel inconvenient to take time to tune in to yourself. Other times, people purposefully repress their emotions to avoid dealing with the pain associated with their underlying issues. The journal prompts in this exercise will awaken your present-moment self. By acknowledging and embracing even potentially distressing feelings, you validate your emotions. This is the first step toward resolving your predicaments.

1. Take a moment to reflect on your day. Did anything happen to make you feel happiness, sadness, anger, frustration, gratitude, doubt, worry, or other feelings? Write down your feelings, and next to each, write down the experience that you think triggered this emotion.

2. What feelings do you have a hard time accepting? Expressing? Why?

3. Challenge yourself to tap into your emotions in real time throughout the rest of your day or week. Write down what you notice about your emotional awareness as you progress.

VISUALIZATION:

My Happy Place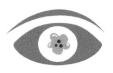

Another way to use visualization is to reduce stress by transporting yourself to a place that brings you peace and joy. When you feel like you can't escape from a tough situation, all you need to do is close your eyes and use the power of your imagination to surround yourself in your happy place. It doesn't matter if you've been to the location in real life, have only seen it in pictures, or are just picturing it for the first time.

1. Sit or lie down. Close your eyes.

2. Take 2 deep breaths.

3. Imagine you are in a place that brings you joy. Look around. Observe everything down to the smallest details to make the visualization come to life in your mind's eye.

4. Listen to the sounds in this peaceful place.

5. Notice the smells. Imagine yourself breathing in slowly and deeply in your visualization, just as you are doing in real life.

6. As you move around, touch anything you can, and notice the textures that you feel.

7. Taste anything possible in your visualization.

8. Continue to observe this happy place using all five senses, and feel the calmness entering into your body.

9. When your timer ends, allow the imagery to gently fade away. Open your eyes.

Lifting the Sky

This technique is a popular Qigong exercise that will energize you when you feel physically or emotionally exhausted and ground you into the present moment, ushering in peace. Qigong is particularly good for balance, posture, and circulation.

1. Stand with your legs a few inches apart, arms by your sides, and your weight evenly distributed between your feet.

2. Open your mouth slightly. Keep your gaze out in front of you.

3. Slowly bring your hands in front of you by your pelvis with your palms facing the ground, fingers spread out and facing each other. Look down at your hands.

4. Keeping this position, raise your arms up in front of you, moving them overhead slowly as you inhale through your nose. Allow your head and gaze to follow the arc of your hands. Bend at the elbows if straight arms are uncomfortable.

5. Once your hands are overhead, palms facing the sky, press up gently as if you are lifting the sky.

6. As you exhale slowly, make a "haa" sound with your breath, and allow your arms to arc downward toward the sides of your body, ending at your starting position.

7. Repeat steps 3 through 6 in a continuous gentle flow until your timer ends.

Affirmations

Affirmations are positive statements of characteristics you want to reinforce about yourself. Affirmations can also refer to characteristics or qualities that you hope to aspire to in the future. You don't have to believe the affirmations when you say them initially. The beauty of repeating affirmations every day is that you change the narrative in your mind from your inner critic's negativity to positive and uplifting self-talk. Over time your mind will start to hold on to these affirmations and believe them, empowering you with confidence and strength.

1. In this moment, what do you need to hear to comfort your-self or boost your sense of self-worth? Write down 5 qualities you want to embody, using the format "I am _____."

2. Try to say these affirmations to yourself each day when you first wake up or at the start or end of your daily mindfulness practices.

3. Every few days, come up with a new list of affirmations to say to yourself.

4. Place your affirmations on sticky notes on your mirror as a visual reminder. You can also type them out as an image saved to your phone to look at every day, especially when you feel sad or unworthy.

4-7-8 Breathing

When you feel a swell of emotions during your pregnancy because of a triggering situation or hormonal changes, it can feel like you are drowning in these emotions. Rather than feeling helpless and succumbing to stress and anxiety, utilize a breathing technique to stop the stress from magnifying. Focusing on your breath moves you from the disruption created by your worries to a calmer state of being. Over time, by slowing your breath, you can access your inner calm more effortlessly.

1. Sit or lie down and close your eyes.

2. Settle into this moment by taking 2 deep breaths. Give yourself permission to let go and decompress. Allow the world around you to gently fade away.

3. Inhale for 4 seconds, taking in as much air as you can.

4. Hold your breath for 7 seconds, keeping count in your mind.

5. Slowly exhale for 8 seconds.

6. Repeat steps 3 through 5, noticing your breath as it moves in and out of your body. Notice how each part of this process makes you feel.

7. When the timer ends, gently open your eyes.

MOVEMENT:
Legs Up

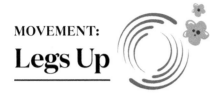

This yoga move is restorative, inviting you to shift from inclinations to perform and instead to receive. Lifting your legs up against a wall also improves circulation, which helps with swollen ankles and legs.

1. Sit next to a wall with your legs outstretched, the left side of your body facing the wall with your left shoulder touching the wall.

2. Place your right elbow on the ground for support. Lift your legs up in the air and move them toward and against the wall while lowering your back to the floor. It might help to use yoga straps, an exercise band, or a towel around your calves to lift your legs up into the air and against the wall.

3. Move your bottom as close to the wall as you can without causing strain on your hamstrings. If your legs feel too stretched, move your bottom further away from the wall to provide relief to the legs.

4. Place your arms on either side of your body, palms facing up to the sky in a receiving pose, opening up your chest.

5. Once settled, take slow, intentional breaths. Witness how your body feels with each breath as it slowly starts to relax.

6. If needed, you can relax from this pose to take a break or to reset. Then repeat steps 2 through 5.

7. To come out of the pose, bend your knees and roll to your side. Use your arms to help push you back up to a seated position.

Not What I Imagined

We've all seen those pictures of the perfectly shaped and pro-portioned pregnant woman who has only gained weight in her belly and exudes that pregnancy glow we are told to expect in our second trimester. The reality is that we are all unique individuals who will have vastly different pregnancy experiences. We will respond to this transformation in a multitude of ways that may not line up with the vision we had in mind. These unmet expectations of perfection, radiance, and vitality can cause feelings of jealousy, shame, anger, and frustration, resulting in disappointment in ourselves and our pregnancy. These journal prompts provide an opportunity to confront deep-rooted feelings and own your truth while providing space to fully accept every part of your extraordinary, unique self.

1. What insecurities do I have about my role as a pregnant person?

2. What expectations of this journey and of myself can I dismantle?

3. Write a short note to yourself embracing who you are at this moment, showering yourself with self-love and compassion.

MEDITATION:
I Am

In this meditation, you will choose one of the affirmations formulated in a previous journal exercise (see page 85). The affirmation will serve as the mantra anchoring you to the present moment while boosting your confidence.

1. Find a comfortable seated or reclined position and close your eyes.

2. Anchor to this moment by witnessing your breath as it moves in and out of your body.

3. Take 3 deep breaths in through your nose and out through your mouth.

4. Allow your breath to settle into a gentle pace.

5. Using one of your affirmations from the journal exercise, repeat this mantra in silence as you inhale. The expansion you feel as you inhale is the words of affirmation filling up your body and mind.

6. As you exhale, notice your body releasing, and imagine the affirmation is nestling deep within your being.

7. Repeat steps 5 and 6 in a slow and methodical manner. With every breath that you take, feel your focus moving inward and your mind shifting toward acceptance of your words of affirmation.

8. When your timer ends, repeat your affirmation one more time. Then wiggle your fingers and toes and gently open your eyes.

Changing Relationships

Being mindful isn't just about self-awareness. It also extends to an awareness of our interactions with others. Life transitions like pregnancy can cause shifts in priorities and availability, making it difficult to maintain existing relationships in their current state. Life changes bring about new perspectives and call on us to evolve. It's okay to admit that you have outgrown some relationships. Attempts to keep life exactly the same as it always was can create frustration and disappointment, causing unnecessary stress. Choose a prompt to answer in your journal:

1. How has pregnancy altered your priorities and availability to interact with your close friends and family? How does this make you feel? How do you think it makes them feel?

2. Life changes can cause strains in relationships. Can you let go of any expectations in your relationships that would help ease the stress?

3. Which relationships light you up and which ones drain you during this season of your life? What shifts can you make in these relationships to prioritize your well-being so you feel energized and happy with the people you choose to spend time with versus feeling depleted or agitated?

I Am Not My Thoughts

Mindfulness gives us agency over our thoughts. Through a nonjudgmental observation of our thoughts as they come and go, we can learn to disassociate from pervasive thoughts and not identify with them. In this meditation, you will label any thoughts that occur as either planning, remembering, criticizing, feeling, or sensation/sound.

1. Find a comfortable seated or reclined position, then close your eyes.

2. Anchor to the present moment by taking 2 deep inhalations through your nose. Make an audible sigh with each exhale.

3. Allow your breath to settle into an intentional pace, and feel your body and mind shifting toward stillness.

4. Observe the breath moving in and out of your body. Notice the rise and fall of your torso in sync with your breath.

5. When a thought occurs, gently acknowledge the thought with grace, and label it as either planning, remembering, criticizing, feeling, sensation, or sound.

6. After observing and labeling the thought, send it on its way and return your focus back to your breath, without judgment of yourself or the thought.

7. Repeat the labeling process every time a thought happens.

8. When the timer ends, open your eyes. Reflect on what type of thought popped up the most in your mind.

BREATHWORK:
Straw Breath

When you have difficult emotions, remember that you can control your breath, which in turn can positively impact your physical, mental, and emotional well-being. The straw breath allows for a greater exchange of oxygen and carbon dioxide, helping when you feel short of breath because of anxiety or limited breathing capacity from a growing belly. Plus, the slower breath instantly triggers a calming effect, easing any mental and emotional distress.

1. In a seated position, place your hands on your belly as a reminder to initiate your breath from this area.

2. Slowly inhale through your nose with your mouth closed.

3. To exhale, purse your lips as if you had a straw in your mouth, and very slowly breathe out through your mouth.

4. As you repeat steps 2 and 3, remember to breathe from your belly in order to fill up with as much air as possible. When you exhale, try to make it longer than your inhale. If it helps, you can keep a mental count of your inhale and exhale.

5. Stay grounded in the present moment by observing how each breath feels as it enters and exits your body.

6. Continue until your timer ends.

Challenge Negativity

Whether we are aware of them or not, we all have beliefs about ourselves that affect our daily life. These beliefs come from memories of how we handled past experiences as well as what people have said about us. These beliefs fuel the narrative of our inner critic, the voice inside our head, judging every move we make and limiting what we allow ourselves to do or be. During pregnancy, emotions can be especially fickle, which can exacerbate the inner critic's influence over your overall disposition and decision-making abilities. Reflect and respond to the following prompts in your journal:

1. What are some limiting beliefs that you have picked up throughout your life? Make a note if someone said this to you or if this was a conclusion drawn from an experience. Challenge the validity of that limiting belief by providing a sentence with evidence of your abilities.

2. What are some things your inner critic has said to you during your pregnancy journey that intensify any feelings of sadness, depression, jealousy, shame, or self-doubt? Remember that it is okay to feel these feelings, and they do not define you as a person. Writing them out ignites awareness, acknowledgment, and a release of your feelings' control over you. Provide countering statements disputing the accuracy of everything you list.

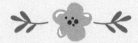

YOU ARE NOT ALONE

If your past involved infertility, miscarriage, or pregnancy loss, becoming pregnant can be a complex blend of elation and apprehension. With 15 to 20 percent of pregnancies ending in miscarriage and one in eight couples having difficulty getting pregnant and requiring assisted reproductive therapy, it is common for people to enter pregnancy with pre-existing emotional pain and trauma. It also means you may have more to unpack in these exercises or need support to do these exercises, as each journey is unique. Remember, the obstacles you faced are not a reflection of your worthiness and ability to be a loving parent. Give yourself grace and take it slow when breaking down the walls of protection you may have built up to guard your heart. Cocoon yourself in an abundance of love and kindness.

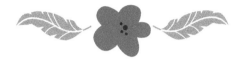

CHAPTER 7

Embrace the Unknown

Stepping into new beginnings means closing one chapter of your life to start a new one. The uncertainty that comes with this kind of change can feel problematic. With pregnancy, there's pressure to embrace the unknown, sometimes when you aren't fully ready to relinquish control of the comforts of your present life. This chapter addresses issues related to the transition that comes with pregnancy and impending parenthood, such as overcoming worry, facing fears, grieving your past, making peace with what's to come, letting go, and opening yourself up to possibilities. Some exercises will teach you techniques to switch up your thinking when you get triggered about the future. Other exercises will reconcile your relationship with the unknown by opening channels of trust, acknowledgment, and acceptance. You'll also train your brain to visualize the challenges of the future so you can imagine using the mindfulness techniques in your toolkit to face obstacles with bravery, strength, and a positive mindset. As you embark on this bold journey into the unknown, extend compassion to yourself and approach each exercise with patience and an open mind. Remain committed to being fully awakened to the present moment, and remind yourself of your desire to navigate what lies ahead with grace and perhaps even a sense of adventure.

5-4-3-2-1

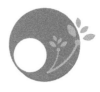

Uncertainty about what will happen in your pregnancy and your future transition into parenthood can breed uncomfortable feelings. When you feel the grips of anxiety or panic taking hold of you, this 5-4-3-2-1 method moves you from being a worrier to a warrior, because tuning in to the sensory aspects of the present moment hits the pause button on your downward spiral and refocuses your attention. An added bonus is that this technique can be done anywhere that you feel triggered. Simply implement this strategy in the heat of the moment and return back to the issue at hand when you feel calmer.

1. What are 5 things you can see? After observing 5 things, take a deep breath.

2. Notice 4 things you can hear in this moment, then take a deep breath.

3. Touch 3 things and notice how they feel. Take another deep breath.

4. Smell 2 things around you. Suggestions if you're struggling to find something to smell: your clothes, your hair.

5. Take one more slow and deep breath in through your nose and exhale slowly out of your mouth.

6. End by saying this mantra: "I am grounded in this moment. I have restored my connection to calm."

Trust the Journey

Opening yourself up to the unknowns of pregnancy means making peace with what's to come, even when you don't know how things will unfold. It requires trust in the process and confidence that you can navigate whatever comes your way. While surrendering to the journey in this meditation and moving out of your comfort zone, you will still feel supported as you cultivate your courage, acceptance, and trust.

1. Sit or lie down. Close your eyes.

2. Turn your attention to your breath. Notice your inhales and exhales, allowing the outside world to gently melt away with each breath.

3. As you focus inward, let each breath awaken your courage. Your courage grows each day with your desire and readiness to meet your baby. Repeat to yourself, "I awaken my courage."

4. Continue observing your breath. Silently repeat these words: "I choose to accept and trust my journey."

5. For the remainder of your meditation, combine the mantras into one. Say it silently with each inhale: "I awaken my courage and choose to accept and trust my journey."

6. With every breath, embrace the unknown with your courageous spirit and trust in yourself.

7. When your timer ends, gently open your eyes.

Honoring Myself through Transitions

The transformation that occurs during pregnancy demonstrates that life is impermanent and we are constantly evolving. During the whirlwind of the gestational period, however, it can be easy to overlook or downplay this important transition. Incorporating mindfulness every day allows you to look at your life through the lens of awareness and embrace the shifts happening internally and externally. Choose one of the following prompts to answer in your journal:

1. Think about your identity and the person you were prior to pregnancy—things you did, things you liked, your personality, your relationships. Honor this version of yourself by remembering some key moments during this time.

2. Think about the person you have become during pregnancy. What has changed? What has remained the same? Take a moment to grieve and celebrate this emotional metamorphosis.

3. Write down the values and characteristics you hope to maintain or develop during your pregnancy and into your role as a parent.

4. Write yourself a short note of encouragement and support as you step out of your comfort zone and into this phase of the unknown. Remind yourself of your bravery and strength and reflect on the promise of chapters yet to unfold.

MOVEMENT:

Seated Side Bend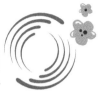

Your growing belly can cause strain on your back as it works hard to balance out the increased weight in the front of your body. This yoga move can alleviate any pregnancy-related backaches you may experience.

1. Sit cross-legged with your arms on either side of your body. Maintain a straight posture with your gaze forward.

2. Ground yourself into this moment by taking 2 deep breaths.

3. Notice your body as it receives the inhale: how it expands and adjusts to the continuous flow of relaxation.

4. On your next inhale, lift your right arm up overhead, fingers pointing to the sky, while placing your left hand on the ground to support you.

5. As you slowly exhale, bend your body toward your left side, allowing your left hand to glide along the floor, away from the body, to help you bend lower. If you are able, allow your left forearm to meet the ground.

6. Hold this seated side bend for a few breaths. Every time you exhale, see if you can increase the stretch just a little bit more.

7. Return back to your starting position.

8. Repeat steps 4 through 7 on the other side, bending toward your right side.

9. Alternate side bends until your timer ends.

20-Week Scan Nerves

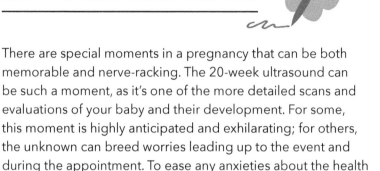

There are special moments in a pregnancy that can be both memorable and nerve-racking. The 20-week ultrasound can be such a moment, as it's one of the more detailed scans and evaluations of your baby and their development. For some, this moment is highly anticipated and exhilarating; for others, the unknown can breed worries leading up to the event and during the appointment. To ease any anxieties about the health of your baby and allow for full enjoyment of this experience, take some time to offload your concerns and switch your thinking. Feel free to use these prompts before any ultrasounds or doctor visits to keep your worries in check. Respond in your journal:

1. What concerns do you have about your upcoming appointment? Acknowledging your feelings is awareness in action and a form of self-compassion.

2. Write out a list of questions to ask the technician or doctor who addresses your concerns. This action gives you some agency over an otherwise uncontrollable process.

3. Although we can't control the thoughts that enter our mind, we do have the power to decide which thoughts we react to and hold on to. Look over your list of concerns and see which ones you can choose to release or reframe from a different perspective.

BREATHWORK:
Letting Go

Exhaling is an activation of release and freedom from constraints. When you're feeling heavy in your mind from mental stress or heavy in your body from physical tension, an elongated exhale can do wonders for decompressing your entire being. With these more pronounced exhales, remind yourself that there is no need to hold on to anything that no longer serves you.

1. Sit or lie down. Close your eyes. Ground yourself into this moment by turning your attention inward.

2. Breathe in slowly and deeply through your nose for 4 seconds.

3. Exhale for a count of 8 seconds. For the first 5 breaths, start with an audible sigh as you exhale, blowing your breath out through your mouth, feeling your shoulders falling away from your ears.

4. Now transition to a regular exhale through your nose, breathing in for 4 seconds and exhaling for 8 seconds.

5. With each exhale, imagine releasing anything that is weighing you down physically or emotionally. None of that needs to be here with you in this present moment.

6. Remind yourself you deserve the opportunity to let go and feel free.

7. When the timer ends, return to the present moment by wiggling your fingers and toes.

Creating a Birthing Mantra

A mantra is a tool for your mind to stay grounded in the present moment. This tool fosters and maintains relaxation. Today, you will examine your perspective of the labor and delivery process and formulate a mantra to harness your strength and keep you focused on delivering your baby amid the physical challenges. Answering the questions below requires introspection, honesty, and vulnerability. It's okay to acknowledge your deepest feelings, even if they don't feel acceptable. Everything you feel is valid. You can also do this if you have a C-section scheduled or want to prepare for that possibility as well.

1. What scares you about the labor and delivery process? Envision the process in depth to access the full spectrum of your concerns.

2. While many of our fears and worries feel out of our control, we do have the power to shift our attention to other aspects of the same situation. Close your eyes and reconsider your birthing process. In the moments when you feel fear bubbling up, replace it with the feeling of love for your baby. Love opens you up to acceptance, strength, joy, and trust.

3. Envision your delivery. Write out the words you need to hear during the process to bolster your confidence, power, and tenacity while easing any fear or discomfort. This will be your birthing mantra. Be sure to share them with your delivery day support system.

Negativity Bias

Our brains are wired to look for danger to ensure our survival. As a result of human evolution, this attention to negativity no longer serves us explicitly for life-and-death situations, but now impacts how we view and respond to many different types of situations. Another aspect of negativity bias is that our brains react and hold on to more negative stimuli than positive stimuli. Knowing this about our natural tendencies gives us the opportunity to use strategies that counteract these behaviors. Answer in your journal:

1. Recall a recent interaction where you fixated on negative aspects of another person, yourself, or the situation. Looking back, were there any positive things that you may have overlooked? Take a moment to reframe the interaction, this time including the positives.

2. In the same way, since we hold on to negative events in our minds more than positive ones, write down some positive things that have happened during your pregnancy journey in order to lock those happy moments in your memory.

3. What are some things that worry you about your pregnancy? How can you reframe your perspective of those negative thoughts?

Waiting Room Toolkit

Although mindfulness is about living in present-moment awareness, it's also about being aware of our tendencies in complicated situations. If you find yourself getting worked up about medical appointments, this exercise takes a proactive approach to dealing with your worries and stress. Here, you'll take advantage of your phone's capabilities to shift you into a state of positivity.

1. Create a folder in your phone's photo or documents section and label it something like "My Happy Place." You can also use a photo book.

2. Add photos of your loved ones that bring you joy.

3. Next, search around the web for some quotes that you find uplifting, supportive, and nourishing. Add them to the folder or book.

4. Add photos of landscapes that bring you peace, such as beaches, rivers, forests, or flowers. These can be pictures from a web search or photos from a vacation.

5. In whatever music app or medium you use, create a playlist of songs that you can listen to while sitting in waiting rooms. Select songs that make you feel happy or relaxed. (Make sure this is a different playlist than the one you made for delivery on page 70.)

6. Access your toolkit whenever you seek a sense of calm during your pregnancy.

Delivering My Baby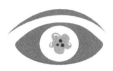

Our imaginations have the capacity to envision a future moment. The purpose of rehearsing this future scenario is not to adhere to a perfect vision of baby's delivery, but to train your brain to operate calmly, even amid obstacles, to reduce present and future anxiety. If your mind has already practiced overcoming challenges, you'll know how to respond if it happens in real life. You can also do this as a C-section visualization, whether it's scheduled or to prepare for that possibility.

1. Lie down. Close your eyes.

2. Allow the world to fade away with each slow breath.

3. Imagine the delivery room, noticing sights, smells, sounds, and textures.

4. Rehearse the process of labor in your mind. Visualize remaining calm and utilize deep-breathing techniques and other mindfulness strategies as you encounter painful contractions, other challenges, or as you await your C-section.

5. See yourself harnessing your inner strength and courage with each deep breath as the contractions come closer together or as you await your C-section.

6. Hear the words your birthing support person is saying to you—your birthing affirmations (see page 79), birthing mantra (see page 102), and/or words of encouragement.

7. Imagine surrendering to the moment with trust and love in those final stages of the birth process.

8. Lock this success, strength, and resilience into your heart and mind.

What Is True?

When our worries become magnified, they can create anxiety. To anchor yourself in the present and stop your mind from ruminating on "what-if" scenarios, challenge the negative narrative you created by using the BEAR (Breathe, Evaluate, Act, Remember) method outlined here. Infusing some calmness and honesty into a situation diffuses the daunting scenario you've created in your mind, allowing you to move forward in a more mindful and less anxious way.

1. **Breathe**: Whenever worries arise, notice them and begin a breathing technique, such as Square Breathing (page 40).

2. **Evaluate**: Once you're feeling calmer, ask yourself, "What do I know in this moment to be true?"

   ✦ Each time, journal your answers to practice challenging the narrative in your mind. By being honest with yourself, you'll find that what's true in this moment might not be a calamity.

   ✦ If you feel it's really a bad situation, ask yourself, "What's the worst that could happen?" Ponder the worst-case scenarios in order to face your fears and give them less power.

3. **Act**: Ask yourself, "Can I do anything about it right now?"

4. **Remember**: Finally, remind yourself, "This hasn't happened, so there's no point in using my mental energy on this. Be present in this moment." Take a deep breath.

Release to Relax

Another way to free yourself from the constraints of physical and emotional stress is to release yourself from expectations and fears. Going through life, we pick up ideas about who we want to be, the best way to exist, and how life should unfold. These thoughts and "shoulds" affect our choices and actions, but they also create expectations that can be unrealistic and harmful. We also hold on to fears about the unknown that prevent us from flourishing and living a life of possibility. Use these journal prompts to let go and open up to life.

1. Make a list of expectations that you have of yourself or others have of you as a human being, as a pregnant person, and as a parent.

2. Cross out the expectations that are not realistic or not in line with your intentions or purpose in life. Circle the ones that align with your truth.

3. As it relates to your pregnancy, what expectations do you have of the process and the birth? Of these expectations that you listed, which ones honor your commitment to being aware of and compassionate with yourself?

4. What fears do you have about life, pregnancy, birth, or other unknowns that you can let go of today?

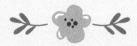

A NOTE ON PERINATAL ANXIETY AND DEPRESSION

Embracing the unknowns of gestation and delivery is a big undertaking for many. Yet for the 10 to 20 percent of women who experience perinatal depression during their pregnancy and/or during the postpartum period, the added uncertainty and hormonal fluctuations can further complicate their experience.

Fortunately, practicing mindfulness cultivates an awareness of your present state, which helps you know when to seek extra help due to overwhelming anxiety and depression. These are common medical conditions; it's important to remember the normalcy of this happening and not feel stigmatized or embarrassed to seek help from your support group or medical team. Assistance is available and can make all the difference. See the Resources section (page 154) for more information.

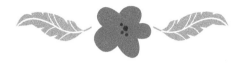

CHAPTER 8

Cultivate a Community of Support

Pregnancy can be a beautiful time of excitement and anticipation, but the rigors can take their toll, especially when carried solely by one individual. During this monumental season of life, it's so helpful to cultivate a community that can celebrate your journey with you. This community can also assist you in alleviating any undue stress from feeling isolated and burdened by the entire responsibility of the pregnancy. If you have a hard time asking for help, some exercises in this chapter will challenge you to reframe your perspective on assistance and give you guidance on how to approach people for help. If you have strained or difficult relationships, there are exercises to channel empathy and directions for opening up lines of communication. You will also create a pregnancy and postpartum proposal so you can delegate tasks to people while establishing boundaries. For the partner exercises in this chapter, the partner refers to anyone who is able to help you, such as a life partner, family member, friend, doula, or birthing coach. If you aren't surrounded by other pregnant people or have a unique situation making it hard to relate to "traditional" pregnancies, there are also tips on how to find a community that's right for you.

JOURNAL:

Receiving Support

During this profound time of transition in which all aspects of your life are changing, it can feel heady and exciting—and it can also feel scary, lonely, and confusing. Having a support system to share in your excitement and lean on for comfort, love, and encouragement can elevate your disposition and overall pregnancy experience. Despite knowing the importance of help, our expectations of our role in pregnancy and the role of others can get in the way of accepting assistance. Answer one or more of the following prompts in your journal to examine your thoughts on aid and dismantle any beliefs that may hinder your ability to build a community of support.

If you aren't in a traditional relationship or have strained relations with family and friends, know that there aren't any rules for how many people you need to have on your side. One good friend can make all the difference. See the Resources on page 154 for suggestions on alternative support systems.

1. Recall a time in your life when you truly felt supported. In what ways were you cared for? What conditions allowed for this to happen?

2. How can you advocate for yourself to receive the support that you need?

3. What can you welcome or let go of in order to feel nurtured?

Establish Boundaries

Opening yourself up to other people's assistance during your pregnancy can radically change your overall experience for the better. Unfortunately, it can also come with some unexpected hassles, such as the overstepping of boundaries. Well-intentioned loved ones can unexpectedly cross the line and invalidate your needs and feelings when they aim to assist through actions or advice. It's essential to create boundaries, or guidelines, to sustain healthy relationships. These boundaries aren't meant to change or control someone; rather, they're meant to establish limits on what you want to receive and to uphold the importance of your needs. Here, you'll formulate and practice communicating boundaries to allow for better understanding.

1. Make a list of boundaries you need in your relationships. Be flexible when establishing boundaries–these may need to change as situations and relationships evolve.

2. Imagine speaking to someone about your need for a boundary. Use "I feel___ when" statements to explain the boundary's importance. Using "I" statements gives you ownership of your feelings without being accusatory toward someone. It prevents defensiveness and promotes open conversation. For example, if a person comes over without calling, you can practice saying "I feel pressured when you come over without calling. I would prefer you ask first so I can make sure I'm available and up for company."

3. As you practice, approach your message with empathy for the other person's perspectives and feelings.

AWARENESS EXERCISE:

Conscious Communication

With all the attention going to you and your growing baby, sometimes partners can get overlooked during the pregnancy. This one-sided prioritization can create feelings of isolation, jealousy, and even discord in the relationship. In this exercise, you will apply mindfulness to your communication to strengthen your relationship with your partner, so you can work as a team collaborating toward a common goal. Taking a few moments to reconnect shows your partner that you value and prioritize them and your relationship. When answering these questions, maintain strong eye contact and validate your partner's responses with gratitude and compassion. Use any of the following prompts to initiate a conversation with your partner, with both of you answering the question(s). It's ideal to do a partner check-in at least once a month during pregnancy.

1. How are you feeling about the pregnancy?

2. What are your stressors at this point, and how can I best support you?

3. What can I do to make you feel more included in the process? (to ask your partner)

4. What can I do to give you a break or help you? (for your partner to ask you)

5. What's one thing I can do for you to make you feel loved and appreciated?

BREATHWORK:
Partnered
Hugging Breath

This exercise is a great way to get your partner or birthing support person involved during pregnancy, labor, or while waiting for your C-section. Physical touch from your partner is beneficial in reducing stress and the perception of pain. Plus, any sort of couples' exercise fosters feelings of usefulness for the partner and support for the pregnant person.

1. Find a comfortable seated position either on the floor, hospital bed, or your birthing area.

2. Have your partner sit behind you, either sitting on their knees, with knees apart if desired, or with their legs straddling your body.

3. Place your hands on your belly. Have your partner wrap their arms around your belly, with your hands touching if possible.

4. Position your faces close together if desired.

5. With your eyes open or closed, together with your partner take a deep breath in through your noses.

6. If possible, try to time your exhales together, breathing out slowly from your noses.

7. Hear the sound of your partner's breath, and observe the touch, movement, and heat of their body against yours.

8. Savor each breath as an opportunity to come together as a cohesive unit.

9. Continue breathing and connecting with one another until the timer ends.

Asking for Help

Recognizing your personal needs and accepting the fact that pregnancy necessitates assistance is the first step toward impactful change regarding support. If you're the type of person who prefers to tackle problems on your own, it can be difficult to ask for help. Reframing the way you look at assistance can give you the push you need to make a bold ask. Instead of viewing your need for help as a flaw or weakness, view your ability to reach out for support as a sign of strength and validation of your self-worth.

1. Make a list of everything that needs to be done in preparation for your baby's arrival. Writing lists can help you organize your thoughts while also releasing them from your mind and onto paper. Write down the person who can take on each task, whether it's you or someone else. Is there a way you can delegate some of your perceived responsibilities to others to lessen your load?

2. Tips for asking someone for help:

   ✦ Do it personally and in private.

   ✦ Use clear communication.

   ✦ Be specific about your needs.

   ✦ Refrain from apologizing for asking, as it adds a layer of shame to the request.

MOVEMENT:
Partner Sacral Press

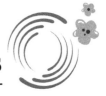

In this exercise, you'll collaborate with your partner or birthing support to bolster your relationship through physical connection. Your partner will press on the lower part of your back to help relieve back pain. This can be done throughout the pregnancy, during labor, or prior to a C-section. It may be helpful to use an exercise ball or cushions to lean your body against to receive the full benefits of this movement.

1. Sit upright on your knees on the floor or bed. Open up your knees for a wide child's pose (see page 59).

2. Have your partner stand or sit behind you.

3. Bending forward from the hips, go as far down as you can, either to the floor or your props. Extend your arms out in front of you up past your ears, or rest them on the sides of your body.

4. Once in position, your partner will place the heel of their hand on your lower back, right above your buttocks, and firmly push in and then downward as if to lengthen your spine.

5. Your partner should place enough pressure to relieve any pain or discomfort, and check how you feel. Stop if you feel pain.

Birthing Proposal

As you move toward your third trimester, you will likely discuss a birthing plan with your obstetrician. Eliminate potential stress from your perceived need to control the situation by thinking of this as a birthing proposal instead of a plan, so it feels more versatile and less rigid. Flexibility is essential, so consider preparing for various scenarios. The advantage of practicing mindfulness prior to labor, delivery, or your C-section is that your flourishing awareness will help you understand your needs in the moment, allowing you to pivot to whichever course of action is required. Do this exercise after you have created at least one draft of your birthing proposal.

1. Review the birthing proposal that you created. Are there any areas for infusing mindfulness into the process of labor and delivery—for example, when you settle into your room, in between contractions, or in the time before your scheduled C-section? Review the exercises in this book and select those you found most effective in reducing stress and increasing calm. Add them to your birthing proposal.

2. Describe the roles of the person or people in your birthing room with regard to keeping you relaxed, present, and supported.

3. Based on the strategies you selected, add the necessary items to your delivery bag list.

Personal Cheerleader

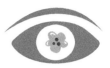

In this visualization, you will use the power of your imagination to be soothed by your personal cheerleader—a person in your life who is typically there to encourage and support you through tough times. This is the person who knows when you need advice, a hug, or a listening ear. You can even use a made-up being as your cheerleader. Your cheerleader can be of great support when you're alone at appointments and need uplifting.

1. Sit or lie down in a comfortable position. Close your eyes.

2. Take 2 deep breaths to anchor to the present moment.

3. Tune in to your current state of being. What uplifting words do you need to hear right now?

4. As you breathe, picture moving from your current location to an empty white space devoid of sound. The only people in this space are you and your personal cheerleader.

5. Smile and give each other a hug, feeling their support enveloping and protecting you.

6. Look into their eyes and feel their love radiating out toward you.

7. Now hear the encouraging words you selected coming out of your cheerleader's mouth. As they repeat these words to you, feel their love enshrouding you and bolstering your spirit.

8. When the timer ends, allow this image to gently fade away, and then open your eyes.

Loving Kindness

This powerful and humbling practice with roots in Buddhism is used to cultivate feelings of love, benevolence, understanding, and forgiveness, first toward yourself and then toward others in your community, including those with whom you may have differences. This meditation can enhance your self-compassion and social relationships through goodwill and empathy.

1. Sit or lie down. Close your eyes.

2. Place a hand over your heart. Ground yourself with 2 deep breaths.

3. While slowly breathing, say the following phrases with deep intention: "May I be happy. May I be healthy. May I be safe. May I live in peace." Take a deep breath after saying these words to yourself to allow these wishes to reverberate throughout your being. Witness how it makes you feel.

4. Imagine someone you love standing in front of you. Look into their eyes, and while deeply breathing, say, "May you be happy. May you be healthy. May you be safe. May you live in peace." Feel the happiness you both experience from this gesture.

5. Repeat step 4 while thinking of an acquaintance, then repeat the step while thinking of someone you have a difficult relationship with. Lastly, extend these wishes to the whole world.

6. When the timer ends, open your eyes and allow this kindness to ripple throughout the rest of your day.

AWARENESS EXERCISE:

A Note of Thanks

A sense of gratitude can boost feelings of appreciation, love, satisfaction, and happiness. It can change your overall outlook, even from the first time you practice gratitude. In this exercise, you'll write a note recognizing someone's kind efforts during your pregnancy. This acknowledgment of kindness can strengthen your relationship with this person as your connection continues to evolve throughout your pregnancy. An expression of thanks can also be a powerful act of forgiveness that can mend a strained relationship. Recognizing someone's efforts exemplifies the positive effects that goodwill has on others and on one's sense of self.

1. Write a letter of gratitude to someone who made a difference to you in a significant way, either through a small act of kindness or a greater effort. Your note can be about something that happened before or during your pregnancy.

2. Make note of the positive impact their efforts had on your life or well-being. You can list any outcome you experienced, big or small.

3. Include a message explaining why they are an important part of your life and journey.

4. Deliver this note in person if possible, so you can experience this joyful moment together.

Shoulder and Back Massage

Much like the other partner exercises in this chapter, this exercise facilitates mindfulness, collaboration, and support; for couples, it can also deepen intimacy. This massage can alleviate any strain felt in the shoulders and back due to the physical demands of pregnancy. If your partner doesn't feel comfortable using their hands for the massage, consider using other tools such as a hand massager or a hard lacrosse ball to soothe your aching muscles. If using hands, their fingers should provide light pressure, and the heel of their hand or a fist can provide a firmer touch. Doing partner massage during pregnancy provides relief and also gives your partner practice for using massage during labor or before a C-section.

1. Create a relaxing environment using your mindfulness music playlist (see page 104) and any scents you've been using for your meditations.

2. Sit in a comfortable position on a chair or bed.

3. Using either hands or a massage tool, have your partner apply firm but comfortable pressure to your shoulders and back, avoiding the spine. Communication of comfort is important to prevent pain or discomfort during the massage and to inform your partner where your body needs more attention.

Postpartum Proposal

A lot of emphasis is placed on pregnancy milestones and birth plans, but it is also essential to mindfully devise a postpartum plan, which we'll call a proposal (since plans can change!). The postpartum period, or "fourth trimester," is an arduous time spent recovering from the delivery of your baby and caring for your newborn. It can be cumbersome to figure out what you need and ask for help once you're in the thick of things, so in this awareness exercise, you'll preempt the hurdles of the fourth trimester by crafting a list of tasks and people who can help you heal.

1. Do you have a hard time asking for help? If so, why? Write out some statements that validate your need for support, love, and care.

2. With the help of your partner, create a list of tasks you might need help with during the postpartum period.

3. Make a list of people in your life who you can depend on, and ask for their help during the postpartum period. Make a plan to ask them ahead of time, laying out specific dates if possible.

4. Assign tasks from your support list to your postpartum support crew.

5. Remind yourself often that it's okay to ask for help. Perhaps keep track of supportive words people said when agreeing to help.

FINDING MY COMMUNITY

For some, you may be the first pregnant person in your network. For others, your road to pregnancy or the pregnancy itself may be different due to your unique circumstances. In any case, you may feel isolated or not seen, heard, or understood. Take stock of how you feel during your pregnancy, making note of what you might need in terms of outside support. This can look like joining a pregnancy group or app, working with a doula, taking a pregnancy course, or searching for your ideal support community on social media. Tune in to your mental and emotional well-being so you can be proactive and find the best support system for your needs. See the Resources on page 154 for suggestions.

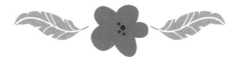

CHAPTER 9

Elevate Simple Daily Habits

We all have our own routine and things we do regularly. Practicing mindfulness in your daily habits can help you grow your ability to be aware and present in all aspects of your life, not just when you sit down to do a 5-minute exercise! By cultivating conscious connections throughout your day, you will gradually build a mindful lifestyle that will benefit you physically, emotionally, and socially. When you are fully present in what you are doing, your actions can translate into feelings of fulfillment, peace, gratitude, and joy.

The exercises in this chapter will encourage evaluation of your daily habits to identify times when you aren't fully present and explore the factors contributing to your disengagement. You'll practice elevating simple tasks that are often taken for granted, like brushing your teeth, eating, walking, standing, sitting, and exercising. Many of these recurring activities are habitual and thus require very little thought, which stifles presence. Doing the exercises in this chapter, on the other hand, will invigorate you and open your eyes to the beauty that surrounds you. Lastly, you will learn the basic principles of how to turn any activity into a mindfulness practice so you can continually infuse awareness into every part of your life.

Autopilot & Multitasking

Before delving into ways to elevate daily habits, it's important to reflect on how you operate throughout your day and find moments that you can optimize with mindfulness. Multitasking, for example, is a habit widely utilized to cope with endless responsibilities. However, working on many things at once actually prevents us from being present in the moment and inhibits our productivity because we're spread too thin and not singularly focused. Many daily tasks are performed on auto-pilot because we've become accustomed to doing them in a certain way. Unfortunately, running on autopilot totally restricts present-moment awareness and prevents any appreciation of what we're doing. As you transition into the busy world of parenthood, the tendencies to use both of these approaches to life can become greater than ever, so pregnancy is the perfect time to practice being fully present in your daily habits.

1. Reflect on today's events. What did you do on autopilot? Did you multitask? How did you feel doing either or both?

2. Are there any daily habits that you always do on autopilot or combine with other tasks?

3. Choose one of those habits to do alone and in a mindful way, and write about how this approach made you feel.

Mindful Toothbrushing

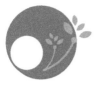

Kick off your day by infusing some mindfulness into your morning rituals, like brushing your teeth. You might typically do this task while you are still in the limbo before fully awakening or against the backdrop of media distractions. In this exercise, you'll practice how to do this seemingly mindless task in a very present way. By infusing mindfulness into your morning routine during pregnancy, you'll know how to put this technique to work during the challenging fourth trimester, when some creative solutions for maintaining routines might be necessary.

1. Before you begin your morning routine, limit your exposure to and interaction with media sources. In doing so, you are extending the stillness from your sleep into your morning for a gradual, peaceful transition into the busyness of life.

2. Take a deep breath to settle into this moment.

3. Before you start brushing your teeth, set an intention (see page 138) for what you would like to embody during your morning ritual.

4. As you brush your teeth, use your intention as your mantra to stay anchored to the present moment. Become aware of your five senses as they relate to brushing your teeth.

5. Once you are done brushing, end with an energizing deep breath. Take your intention with you so you can continue to embody it during the rest of your day.

MEDITATION:
Walking Mindfully

Another daily activity that we take for granted and often infuse with multitasking is going for a walk. Whether you're taking a quick walk from your car to the store or a longer walk meant for relaxation and exercise, distractions and autopilot behaviors can prevent you from witnessing your surroundings. For the purposes of this exercise, you'll go on a quick walk that will be elevated mindfully through sensory observation. If walking isn't an option for you, consider another physical movement that you often find yourself multitasking with.

1. Set your phone timer and put the phone on airplane mode, placing it in your pocket or purse to prevent distractions.

2. As you start walking, take long, slow inhales and exhales through your nose. Notice how the breath is entering and exiting your body.

3. Soften your body with each exhale.

4. Start by tuning in to your sense of sight. Look all around you and take everything in. Don't forget to look up and appreciate what's above you. Enjoy the visual splendor unfolding before your eyes with every step you take.

5. Next, listen to the sounds and notice the scents around you. As you walk, try to take in both the obvious and subtle sounds and smells to fully experience the present moment.

6. Breathe in gratitude for this awakened experience.

Mindful Eating

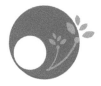

During different stages of pregnancy, it can be difficult to eat because of nausea or indigestion. When you have the ability and inclination to eat, observe the process of how you eat over the course of a few meals. Are you eating while doing something else, like working or looking at social media? How about the rate at which you are eating? How did you feel after you ate? Satisfied? Rushed? Notice if you feel any physical effects from the manner in which you ate. After this mindful observation of your eating habits, amplify your eating process using the following mealtime mindfulness tips.

If you have trauma in this area, some additional support for this exercise may help. You know yourself the best.

1. Sit with your plate of food in an area free from distractions such as work or media.

2. As you pick up your utensil, take a moment to visually savor what you are about to eat.

3. Take your first bite and put your utensil back down. Chew slowly to taste your food. Observe the textures and smells. Notice how the food makes you feel.

4. Continue to take each subsequent bite as directed in step 3 until your entire meal is done.

5. How did it feel to eat in this manner? Journal about your experience.

JOURNAL:
Life Audit
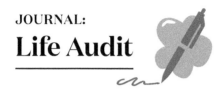

In thinking about your daily routines and how you can revamp your life with awareness, a necessary step is to evaluate any opportunities for growth. The more you practice being mindful in all aspects of your life, the more you'll start to notice an increase in overall clarity. Your present-moment observations will enable you to make small changes in your daily functioning that will make way for meaningful transformation. As you undertake the more obvious preparations for parenthood, conducting this "life audit" can strengthen your groundwork for becoming a better prepared parent. Choose one or more of the following prompts to answer in your journal or to contemplate.

1. Reflect upon your typical day, or think about yesterday. What distractions did you face that prevented you from doing things that needed to get done?

2. Do you procrastinate? What excuses do you make? Is there a pattern in this process?

3. What drains your energy? Are there things or people in your life that deplete you instead of nourishing you? Is there a way to replace these interactions with more of what fulfills you?

Finding Time for Myself

Do you feel like you don't have enough time or plenty of time? Are you time-poor or time-abundant? Those who feel they lack time in the day feel stressed. Conversely, those who feel they have time on their side feel happier. There are simple ways to reframe your perspective and use time to your advantage. In a world that values productivity, it can be difficult to give merit to the idea of stillness. Please remember that there's tremendous value in taking time to disconnect from the world and reconnect with yourself. Choose one of the following exercises that resonates with you.

1. To decrease your stress over lack of time, block off periods for work and leisure in your calendar. Seeing your time planned over a week can ease your worries and make it easier to relax during your scheduled self-care moments. Be realistic when blocking your time. Unreasonable expectations can also cause stress.

2. When looking at your task list, define levels of urgency. Select 3 things a day from your urgent list to tackle.

3. Increase the free time you have by setting up systems that give you more time, like meal prepping, automatic bill payment, delegating, etc.

MOVEMENT:
Mindful Exercise

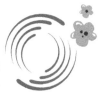

During exercise, it's common to get distracted by the activity, background music, or other stimuli. However, exercise is a beneficial and important time to tune in to your body, observe how it feels, and make sure you are staying safe. It's also highly effective to mindfully pair your breath with your movement. For example, exhaling can help you stretch further into a position or help you lift a weight. In this exercise, you will practice being mindful while you perform a bridge pose. This yoga pose strengthens the leg muscles and promotes flexibility in the back and shoulders.

1. Lie on your back, knees bent, arms by your sides, chest open, and shoulders pressed down and away from your ears. Your feet should be flat and grounded, with your fingertips grazing your heels.

2. Inhale deeply.

3. As you exhale, press your feet against the floor, tighten your glutes (buttocks) and core (belly) muscles, and lift from your hips, aiming your pelvis toward the sky.

4. Continue squeezing your glutes at the top of your bridge position. Take 5 deep breaths as you hold this pose, observing your body and your breath.

5. Slowly release your body down to your starting position. Repeat steps 2 through 4 until your timer ends, resting as long as you need between each repetition.

AWARENESS EXERCISE:

Elevated Self-Care

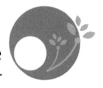

Self-care is a valuable tool in maintaining well-being, espe-cially during pregnancy and the postpartum period. Self-care is often looked upon as a luxury or something that requires a lot of money, time, or products. It isn't. Perhaps taking the time to care for oneself feels selfish. It *definitely* isn't. If you feel this way, the first step in revamping your outlook on self-care is to reframe your perspective. Instead, view such activities as an essential step in maintaining physical, mental, and emo-tional well-being. Use these prompts and tips to evaluate your self-care practices and amplify them with mindful intention.

1. Do you prioritize your well-being over other parts of your life, such as work, friends, or home tasks? If this does not happen on a consistent basis, what gets in the way?

2. When you think about caring for yourself and prioritizing your well-being, what feelings or thoughts come to mind?

3. Before you begin any self-care activity, set an intention (see page 138) for your purpose. How do you want to feel during and after this wellness practice?

4. As you proceed through your self-care time, establish some affirmations to support why you are doing this activity. For example, "I am worthy. I deserve restoration and healing." Repeat it in your mind throughout your self-care time.

Rooted to the Ground

With all the standing you do on a daily basis, it's to your benefit to strengthen this simple act, especially since pregnancy can cause imbalance as the belly grows. The feet are our first point of connection to the earth beneath us. They root us to the ground, from which we base our stability and power. In this exercise, you'll practice strengthening your standing position so you can eventually apply this foot activation whenever you exercise or walk. This awareness will help you stand firm as your center of gravity continues to change throughout pregnancy.

If standing is not an option for you, consider other connections to the ground you can make with your body.

1. Stand with your feet shoulder-width apart.

2. Face forward. Relax your shoulders, arms, and face.

3. Lift your toes, spread them out, and place them firmly on the ground.

4. Feel each toe and the four corners of your feet against the floor while trying to lift your arches.

5. Feel the power generated from your feet and move it upward to the rest of your body by squeezing your leg muscles, glutes, pelvic floor muscles, and core.

6. Once in this position of strength, take deep intentional breaths and observe the power your body has created. Check in with your connection to the ground. Rest and reactivate muscles as needed.

MEDITATION:

Heart's Desire

As we move through life running on autopilot, multitasking, and feeling starved for time, we can lose our connection to our sense of self and our needs. To regain this connection, it's essential to hit the pause button during the day and take a moment to reconnect with our heart's desire. In this exercise, you'll elevate your meditation by pondering a deep question.

1. Lie down using props for comfort. Spread your arms out in a T formation. As you extend your arms out, feel your chest opening up. Allow for a small curve in your back to open your chest up further if you like.

2. Close your eyes.

3. Inhale deeply and feel the breath expanding in the space that you created in your chest.

4. Exhale to release any tension in your body or mind.

5. Continue to notice the breath as it moves through this openness you've created in your body.

6. Ask yourself, "What does my heart truly desire right now?" Embrace this opportunity to look inward honestly. Surrender to whatever comes to the surface. There's no need to force anything. Just allow things to flow organically.

7. When the timer ends, open your eyes.

Mindful Nesting

As you progress into late pregnancy, you might feel this internal need to start preparing your environment for the arrival of your baby—that's "nesting." Infuse mindfulness into this special time so your environment enhances your overall well-being, especially since you'll be spending a lot of time in this space. Evaluate how the room makes you feel once you're done decorating. You may need to take time away from the space after redecorating and revisit it later to get a fresh perspective. Apply these same tips to the rest of your living space to transform your entire home into a serene sanctuary. Select an exercise below to kick-start your mindful nesting.

1. Create a mood board by making a list of calming colors and textures that you would like to use. Colors and textures can contribute to the overall vibe of the room, softening and enlivening your space. Think about how you can add these elements to your space.

2. Since babies require a lot of equipment, consider what you can put in baskets, drawers, or cabinets to remove some of the clutter from your vision.

3. Lighting affects mood. Take time to assess the lighting in your living space. Consider how you can choose soft light, preferably with a dimmer, which also helps a baby transition into and out of the dark after all those months spent in your cozy, dim womb.

BREATHWORK:
Seated Serenity

You'll spend a lot of time feeding and soothing your baby from the comforts of your bed or nursery chair. It can be easy to take all this sitting for granted, yet these times can be turned into mindful moments that strengthen your connection with your child. Practice this seated breath now so you'll remember how to use it during those future feeding sessions in your postpartum period, when you'll be craving a mix of energy and calm.

1. Sit in a relaxed but purposeful position: straight back with shoulders pulled back.

2. Hold a pillow in your arms to simulate the feel of a baby.

3. Use props to support your body if needed.

4. Close your eyes.

5. If you're in a rocking chair or glider, begin to slowly rock back and forth.

6. Take 2 deep breaths, releasing audible sighs. Settle into the moment.

7. Continue taking healing breaths while allowing the outside world to melt away.

8. Let your inhale fill you with energizing oxygen while your exhale releases stress to make room for relaxation.

9. Continue this pattern of renewal via your inhale and exhale until the timer ends.

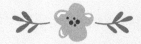

HOW TO TURN
ANYTHING INTO A
MINDFULNESS EXERCISE

As you have undoubtedly discovered from the exercises in this chapter, it is absolutely possible to turn any seemingly ordinary activity into an eye-opening, mindful experience. Recall that the ultimate goal is to eventually establish mindfulness as the overall foundation upon which you live. Here are some tips to remember when applying mindfulness to any activity:

✦ Remove other distractions when possible.

✦ Focus on the moment or activity by observing all the details, tuning in to your five senses.

✦ Slow down the steps involved.

✦ If you find your mind wandering, gently acknowledge the distraction without judgment. Allow the thought to float gently out of your mind, knowing you can return to it later.

✦ Savor each moment with gratitude.

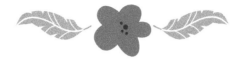

CHAPTER 10

Morning Moments & Evening Wind-Downs

Starting each day with intention and mindful moments provides a gentle transition from a state of rest into the busyness of your day. If you are observant, calm, grateful, and methodical in the morning, you'll set a wonderful tone and pace for your daily activities. You'll also find some exercises in this chapter that encourage revitalization through gentle movement. These activities will provide a boost of energy for those moments in your pregnancy when you feel sluggish.

Of equal importance to how you begin your day is how you end it. The second half of this chapter focuses on evening relaxation rituals, which can be particularly helpful for pregnant women who experience insomnia. First, you will examine your current regimen to determine areas for improving your sleep hygiene. Then, you will practice several strategies to help you settle your mind, relax your body, and ultimately ease into deep, restorative sleep. At the end of the chapter, you'll find tips on how to create a longer mindfulness session whenever you feel ready to take your practice to the next level.

MEDITATION:

Setting an Intention

Jump-start your morning by setting an intention that offers a guiding principle or road map for your day. Different from a goal that is a specific thing that you want to achieve, an intention is your commitment to how you will act or the characteristics you want to embody throughout your day. Reaffirming your intention throughout your day can ultimately help you achieve your goals. For example, you can set a morning intention of patience, which can help you in your interactions with others. As you go through your day, every time you take a deep breath, recall the intention you set in the morning to redirect you back onto your intended path.

1. When you first wake up, sit up in bed, keeping your eyes closed.

2. Take a deep inhale to welcome the new day into your being.

3. Exhale slowly to set the tone for a calm and productive day.

4. Repeat steps 2 and 3 two more times.

5. Now call to mind an intention for your day.

6. On your next inhale, say this intention to yourself.

7. Exhale slowly.

8. Repeat steps 6 and 7 two more times.

9. Breathe deeply until your timer ends.

JOURNAL:
Waking Up Slowly

Do you wake up and quickly run through your mental agenda while your body lazily catches up? Perhaps you immediately grab your phone to check emails, social media, or the news. To dramatically alter your wake-up routine and set a mindful and calm tone for your day, take the time to notice your surroundings and channel appreciation. By starting with an intentional morning moment, you'll ease into your transition from sleepiness to wakefulness, honoring your desire to be calmly aware. Either write in your journal or simply observe, making note of it in your mind. If journaling, keep your notebook next to your bed so it's right there, ready for you.

1. Upon waking up, slowly adjust yourself into a comfortable seated position.

2. Take 2 slow, deep breaths in and out through your nose to welcome the new day into your being. Allow each breath to gradually increase your vitality.

3. Look around and observe 5 things, using as many senses as possible when selecting and witnessing these five things. Try to choose different things each day you do this exercise.

4. End with a moment of appreciation for the day to come.

Sun Salutation

Kick-start your day on an uplifting note by performing some gentle movement to get your blood flowing, your body working, and vibrant energy flowing through you. This yoga move is modified from the original version to account for your growing belly, but it's best done in the first trimester and the beginning of the second unless you are comfortable with these movements later in your pregnancy.

1. Stand with your feet hip-distance apart, arms by your sides.

2. Bring your hands together in a prayer position at your heart center. Exhale.

3. As you inhale, bring your arms outward from the prayer position into a T, and then continue circling them upward to overhead, meeting your palms together, fingertips to the sky.

4. Exhale while bringing your hands back down toward your heart center. Hinge at the hips to bend forward, arms dangling toward the floor, knees with a slight bend.

5. Inhale as you lift your head up, bringing your torso up slightly to a flat-back position.

6. Exhale. Bend forward, placing both palms firmly rooted on the ground, bringing each foot back to extend the body in a plank position.

7. Inhale while bending one knee at a time toward the ground, as the opposite heel reaches back to initiate a deep calf stretch.

8. Exhale. Bend at your knees and slowly walk your hands toward your feet. Gradually roll up to a standing position.

9. Repeat as time permits.

Thankful Heart

Practicing gratitude is a powerful technique that can shift your mindset from negativity to positivity and from lack to abundance. Incorporating gratitude into your daily routine results in a multitude of physical, emotional, and social benefits that include decreased stress, increased satisfaction and peace, enhanced emotional awareness, improved mood, less perceived pain, greater empathy, and stronger relationships. By weaving a daily gratitude practice into your morning or evening routine, you'll facilitate a therapeutic pause in your day for reflection that cultivates happiness and contentment. When listing your "gratitudes," remember that they can be big or small things.

1. List 5 gratitudes when you wake up. This will set a positive tone for the rest of your day.

2. List 5 gratitudes before bed. This offers a moment of gentle reflection on your day's events. It also trains your brain to look for the good things that happen in life versus ruminating over negative events. Finally, it fosters appreciation and calm, which aids in restful sleep.

MEDITATION:

Energy Barrier

The time you have when you first wake up is a precious window of opportunity for self-care. It's a beautiful moment to savor before beginning your day, when life quickly becomes distracting, draining, or complicated. In this meditation, you will create an imaginary force field around yourself to protect against any negativity that you may encounter that day.

1. Sit or lie down. Close your eyes.

2. Settle into this peaceful moment by taking 2 deep breaths in and out through your nose.

3. Allow the stillness of the morning to envelop you in its calm.

4. Inhale deeply through your nose.

5. As you exhale slowly through your mouth, imagine you're blowing out a circle of protection around your entire body. Visualize a bright, powerful circle of energy surrounding your body.

6. Repeat steps 4 and 5. When you blow out your next energy barrier, visualize another circle of light around the first force field.

7. With every breath and barrier you create, know that you are protecting yourself from the stressors of the coming day. You do not need to take on other people's energy or stress. Know that with every breath, you create a formidable barrier that prevents negativity from penetrating your being.

MOVEMENT:

Squat

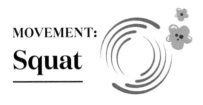

The squat is a fantastic exercise that works many muscles in your body and strengthens your hips, preparing you for birth. You can hold on to something sturdy for extra stability as you do this exercise, if desired.

1. Begin in a standing position, feet hip-distance apart, toes turned slightly outward to your comfort.

2. Firmly plant the bottoms of your feet into the ground (see page 132 for technique).

3. Anchor yourself in the moment by taking a deep breath in and out of your nose.

4. Inhale. Place your hands in a prayer position at your heart center or raise your arms overhead past your ears.

5. Exhale as you slowly squat, keeping your weight back. Bend at your knees, keeping your back flat, chest open, gaze straight ahead, and thighs almost parallel to the ground. Stop lowering when it feels right to you.

6. Either hold this position as you breathe deeply for a few breaths or pulse gently up and down a few inches a few times.

7. Stand up to your starting position by pushing from your heels. Rest as needed.

8. Repeat steps 4 through 8 until your timer ends. Do not push yourself to the point of discomfort. Stop if you feel any pain.

AWARENESS EXERCISE:

Sleep Hygiene

Pregnancy can cause insomnia during the first and third trimester due to stress or discomfort from physical side effects. With sleep during pregnancy already being so problematic, it's a good time to evaluate your sleep hygiene, or your habits for getting a good night's rest. Quality sleep depends on your daily routines as well as the immediate activities right before you get into bed. Follow these prompts to mindfully create a sleep routine.

1. Consider things you currently do before bed or throughout your day that might interfere with quality rest.

2. Choose a consistent time frame for bed.

3. Think about items you can add to your room and bed to create a cozier environment. Ideas might include a diffuser, body pillow, eye mask, etc.

4. Try the following tips for sleep improvement. Make notes of what works and what doesn't. Test out one thing at a time as opposed to changing everything at once.

    ✦ Stop blue light screens an hour before bed.

    ✦ Stop drinking and eating a couple of hours before bed.

    ✦ Put your phone on silent mode and/or leave it in another room.

    ✦ Add a mindfulness exercise you learned to your sleep routine, such as breathing exercises, meditation, visualization, or gratitude.

What Brings Me Joy?

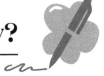

If you've had a tough day or feel worried about something, it can be difficult to stop negative thoughts. A brooding mind can prevent you from falling asleep. One strategy for releasing negativity is to shift toward uplifting and productive thoughts, such as identifying what brings you joy. Much like the art of gratitude, writing down or recalling joyful moments from your day can elicit happiness and appreciation. Once in this positive frame of mind, your brain and body are better able to relax and rest. Answer any of the following prompts to cultivate joy.

1. Who makes you happy through inspiration, support, or camaraderie?

2. What things or events made you feel joyful today?

3. Did you witness any joyful moments that happened to other people?

4. If you had a really bad day and find it difficult to pinpoint anything that was joyful, reflect on previous days this week to find a moment that made you smile. Relive that moment in your mind. Remember every aspect of that experience in order to fully conjure the happiness you felt at that time. This reminds us that life is fluid, and bad moments don't last forever.

BREATHWORK:
Humming Breath

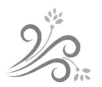

Incorporating breathwork into your sleep ritual can help you unwind and ease you into deeper, more restorative sleep. In this breathing exercise, you'll activate your relaxation response, and the sound that your breath makes can add a soothing, hypnotic component to the experience. You don't need a timer for this exercise.

1. Prepare your environment for sleep, following your other wind-down rituals.

2. Lie down in bed and close your eyes.

3. Gently welcome 2 deep breaths into your being. Feel your body melting into the bed with each exhale and the happenings of the day becoming a distant memory.

4. Inhale steadily through your nose.

5. To exhale, keep your mouth closed and make a soft humming sound in your throat similar to the sound of a buzzing bee. The exhale is happening as you make this humming sound. Extend the humming exhale as long as you can.

6. On your next breath, inhale through your nose, and exhale through your nose without a humming sound.

7. Alternate between the humming breath and regular breath by repeating steps 4 through 6.

8. Feel the vibration of the hum massaging your throat and lulling you into a state of ease.

9. Continue until you fall asleep or feel ready to transition into a restful slumber.

AWARENESS EXERCISE:

Settling My Mind

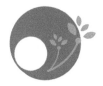

A racing or preoccupied mind can deter relaxation and cause sleep issues. One calming strategy is to reflect on your day and review your schedule and list of tasks for tomorrow. The goal is to give your mind the space and comfort to think and plan versus fighting to suppress it. Try to do this before your other sleep routine habits.

1. What happened today that you are still ruminating over? Write it down or audio-record yourself detailing the experience.

2. Once you're done with your recap, take a deep breath. Remind yourself, "Those moments are all done and in my past. There's no need to bring them with me to bed."

3. Next, take a look at your schedule, if you have it written down somewhere or on your phone. If you don't, write down tomorrow's main events, and organize your day to ease your mind of future worries.

4. Then remind yourself, "Tomorrow is all set. I can let go of future thinking so I can get some rest."

Bedtime Countdown

Another way to transition into a restful state and set the stage for restorative sleep is to use a counted breathing technique. By focusing your mind on your breath and the act of counting, you shift your mind from overpowering thoughts to the present moment while activating your relaxation response. Do this practice once you've completed all of your nighttime routines and any other mindfulness exercises that you do at night. The goal is to lull you into a state of tranquility, making it easier to fall asleep afterward. You don't need a timer for this exercise.

1. Adjust your environment with the necessary sleep aids and calming accessories before settling into bed.

2. Lie down comfortably in bed.

3. Close your eyes and take 5 deep breaths to anchor to this moment of ease. As you exhale, let go of your day. Release any stress weighing on your mind or body and feel your body melting into your bed.

4. Begin your countdown by inhaling and saying, "I surrender to stillness."

5. Exhale and say "20."

6. Repeat steps 4 and 5, counting down from 19 to 1.

7. If you lose track, simply begin again at 20.

MEDITATION:
Gratitude

In this exercise, you'll combine the healing art of meditation with gratitude for an effective practice to foster positivity, calm, and appreciation. If done in the morning, this meditation jump-starts your gratitude awareness so you can better observe anything good that happens throughout your day. If done in the evening or before bed, this practice facilitates mindful contemplation of your day, inviting calm into your being, which can improve sleep quality.

1. Sit or lie down. Close your eyes.

2. With each deep breath, allow your body to soften.

3. Allow the outside world to fade away and feel your body decompress with each breath. This time is just for you.

4. Call to mind something you are grateful for today. On your next inhale, breathe in the joy that you feel from this gratitude, and allow it to fill up your being with happiness. Then slowly exhale.

5. Repeat step 4 four more times, using different gratitudes each time.

6. Before you end your meditation, extend gratitude to yourself for taking the time to prioritize your wellness.

7. End your meditation by taking 2 deep breaths, allowing the peace and joy created by your gratitude to ripple throughout your entire being.

CREATING A
LONGER RITUAL

Whether you've tried only a few exercises in the book or completed nearly every exercise, be proud of yourself for trying something new! By venturing out of your comfort zone, you learned new techniques to add to your self-care toolkit. Ready to extend your mindfulness sessions? Here are some ideas for doing so:

✦ Start by adding an extra minute to your timer. Ease yourself into a longer practice to make it approachable and sustainable.

✦ Add an intention (see page 138) to the beginning of your practice.

✦ List some gratitudes at the end of your practice to spark happiness and appreciation.

✦ Add a breathing technique before a meditation, movement, or journaling session to ground it to the present and invoke peace into your being.

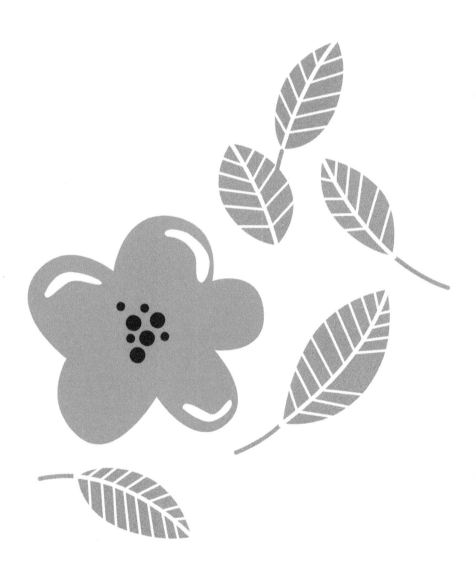

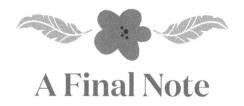

A Final Note

Congratulations on completing this mindfulness guide! The exercises you did laid the groundwork for approaching pregnancy from a lens of awareness to cultivate calm, clarity, and appreciation. You now have the depth of knowledge, framework, and tools to implement a variety of strategies to combat stress, anxiety, exhaustion, discomfort, isolation, sadness, fear, and more. These exercises will continue to be beneficial during your postpartum period and parenthood. Make a plan to revisit the practices in this book, and tailor them to your evolving needs. As your level of comfort with mindfulness flourishes, dare to experiment with your conscious connections while keeping the following tips in mind:

✦ Be flexible with your approach.

✦ Tune in to yourself.

✦ Be honest about what you really need.

✦ Always extend grace, compassion, and love to yourself.

✦ If you get sidetracked by thoughts, acknowledge the distraction without judgment upon yourself or the thought. You don't have to identify with the thought. Give yourself permission to let it go.

✦ Release the weight of expectations on the process and outcome. Instead, surrender to the experience and open yourself up to possibilities, expansion, and awakening.

✦ Focus on the journey, not the destination.

Remember, mindfulness can be applied to any aspect of your life. The more you embed mindfulness into various activities in your daily life, the more you awaken to the beauty of the world around you and further develop your mindful lifestyle.

I hope this discovery has enhanced your overall pregnancy experience, filling you with gratitude, peace, confidence, and joy. Thank you for taking this journey of exploration and trusting yourself and the process of mindful awakening.

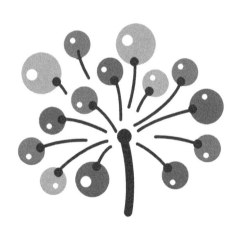

Resources

Apps

Peanut
A safe space to connect with other women about fertility, pregnancy, and motherhood.

What to Expect
Personalized content based on your due date, and access to an online community and other supportive resources.

Books

Mindfulness Journal for Parents: Prompts and Practices to Stay Calm, Present, and Connected by Josephine Atluri

The Feel-Good Pregnancy Cookbook: 100 Nutritious and Delicious Recipes for a Healthy 9 Months and Beyond by Ryann Kipping RDN, CLEC

The First-Time Mom's Pregnancy Journal: Monthly Checklists, Activities & Journal Prompts by Aubrey Grossen

We're Pregnant! The First-Time Dad's Pregnancy Handbook by Adrian Kulp

Websites

Mental Health America
MHAnational.org
Mental health screening tools, directory of support groups, and mental health providers in your area.

Mindful Pregnancy Class
MindfulPregnancyClass.com
Find many of the exercises in this book in audio and video format for extra guidance.

Motherly
Mother.ly
Articles and online classes on pregnancy and motherhood.

Postpartum Support International
Postpartum.net
Essential information on perinatal mood and anxiety disorders, including an online provider directory and resources.

Robyn
WeAreRobyn.co
Find and book parental wellness specialists for pregnancy and parenting, and find therapists for perinatal depression.

The Bump
TheBump.com
Pregnancy and parenting advice, registry, and online community.

The Motherhood Center
TheMotherhoodCenter.com
Virtual mental health center specializing in treating pregnant and postpartum moms with mood and anxiety disorders.

Podcasts

Atluri, Josephine. *Responding to Life: Talking Health, Fertility & Parenthood.*

Leachman, Alexia. *Fear Free Childbirth Podcast.*

Lozada, Adriana. *Birthful.*

Spears, Nina. *Chick Chat: The Baby Chick Podcast.*

Warren, Jay. *Healthy Births, Happy Babies.*

References

Ackerman, Courtney E. "MBSR: 25 Mindfulness-Based Stress Reduction Exercises and Courses." *Positive Psychology*. Accessed October 3, 2021. PositivePsychology.com/mindfulness-based -stress-reduction-mbsr.

Cascio, Christopher N., Matthew Brook O'Donnell, Francis J. Tinney, Matthew D. Lieberman, Shelley E. Taylor, Victor J. Strecher, and Emily B. Falk. "Self-Affirmation Activates Brain Systems Associated with Self-Related Processing and Reward and Is Reinforced by Future Orientation." *Social Cognitive and Affective Neuroscience* 11, no. 4 (April 2016): 621–29. doi:10.1093/scan/nsv136.

Chowdhury, Madhuleena R. "The Neuroscience of Gratitude and How It Affects Anxiety and Grief." *Positive Psychology*. Accessed October 19, 2021. PositivePsychology.com /neuroscience-of-gratitude.

Clear, James. *Atomic Habits: Tiny Changes, Remarkable Results: An Easy & Proven Way to Build Good Habits & Break Bad Ones.* New York: Avery, 2018.

Dhillon, Anjulie, Elizabeth Sparkes, and Rui V. Duarte. "Mindfulness-Based Interventions During Pregnancy: A Systematic Review and Meta-Analysis." *Mindfulness* 8 (April 2017): 1421–37. doi:10.1007/s12671-017-0726-x.

Fox, Kieran C.R., Savannah Nijeboer, Matthew L. Dixon, James L. Floman, Melissa Ellamil, Samuel P. Rumak, Peter Sedlmeier, and Kalina Christoff. "Is Meditation Associated with Altered Brain Structure? A Systematic Review and Meta-Analysis of Morphometric Neuroimaging in Meditation Practitioners." *Neuroscience & Biobehavioral Reviews* 43 (June 2014): 48–73. doi:10.1016/j.neubiorev.2014.03.016.

Herndon, Jaime, MS, MPH, MFA. "Having Anxiety vs. Feeling Anxious: What's the Difference?" *Healthline*. August 9, 2021. Healthline.com/health/anxiety/anxiety-vs-anxious#examples.

Madore, Kevin P., and Anthony D. Wagner. "Multicosts of Multitasking." *Cerebrum* 2019 (April 2019). NCBI.NLM.NIH.gov /pmc/articles/PMC7075496.

March of Dimes. "Stress and Pregnancy." Accessed September 27, 2021. MarchOfDimes.org/complications/stress-and -pregnancy.aspx.

MBCT.com. "Homepage." Accessed September 15, 2021. MBCT.com.

Neal, David T., Wendy Wood, and Jeffrey Quinn. "Habits—A Repeat Performance." *Current Directions in Psychological Science* 15, no. 4 (August 2006): 198–202. doi:10.1111/j.1467 -8721.2006.00435.x.

Resolve. "Medical Conditions." Accessed October 27, 2021. Resolve.org/infertility-101/medical-conditions.

Resolve. "Multiple Miscarriage." Accessed October 27, 2021. Resolve.org/infertility-101/medical-conditions /multiple-miscarriage.

Sayres Van Niel, Maureen, and Jennifer L. Payne. "Perinatal Depression: A Review." *Cleveland Clinic Journal of Medicine* 87, no. 5 (May2020): 273–77. doi:10.3949/ccjm.87a.19054.

Sriboonpimsuay, Wanlapa. 2011. "Meditation for Preterm Birth Prevention: A Randomized Controlled Trial in Udonthani, Thailand." *International Journal of Public Health Research* 1, no. 1 (September 2011): 31–39. Spaj.ukm.my/ijphr/index.php /ijphr/article/view/121.

Xiao, Qianguo, Caizhen Yue, Weijie He, and Jia-yuan Yu. "The Mindful Self: A Mindfulness-Enlightened Self-View." *Frontiers in Psychology* 8 (October 2017): 17–52. doi:10.3389/fpsyg.2017 .01752.

Index

J

K

L

M

S

T

U

V

W

Y

Acknowledgments

Thank you,

Pramod, for your unyielding support and love. You make my heart sing.

Joe and Carol, my parents, for modeling hard work.

Rajendra and Indira, my in-laws, for demonstrating benevolence.

Jaiden, Malena, Mateo, Deion, Dante, Josephine, and Juliette, my masterpieces. Thanks for inspiring me. Love you all.

Suze Yalof Schwartz, and davidji, my mentors, for your guidance.

Farita Reyes Social Media, Light Years Ahead PR, Kristen Mann Design, Allysa Sing, The Network Studios, Good Monday Creative, Patty, Elizabeth, Joelle, for your support during this second book.

About the Author

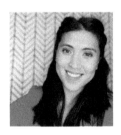

Josephine Atluri is an expert in meditation and mindfulness, helping thousands of people overcome adversity to find joy. A University of Chicago graduate, Josephine coupled her consulting background with her passion for wellness to become certified as a meditation coach. Her experience creating her family of seven children via IVF, adoption, and surrogacy inspires her work as a sought-after fertility and parenting mindfulness coach. She is the author of the highly rated book *Mindfulness Journal for Parents*. Josephine hosts the podcast *Responding to Life: Talking Health, Fertility & Parenthood*. Her expertise has been featured in *MindBodyGreen*, *Motherly*, *Prevention*, and *Woman's Day*.

CPSIA information can be obtained
at www.ICGtesting.com
Printed in the USA
LVHW020457050522
717995LV00020B/987